Anaesthesia: A Very Short Introduction

Very Short Introductions available now:

ACCOUNTING Christopher Nobes
ADVERTISING Winston Fletcher
AFRICAN AMERICAN RELIGION
    Eddie S. Glaude Jr
AFRICAN HISTORY
    John Parker and Richard Rathbone
AFRICAN RELIGIONS Jacob K. Olupona
AGNOSTICISM Robin Le Poidevin
AGRICULTURE Paul Brassley and
    Richard Soffe
ALEXANDER THE GREAT Hugh Bowden
ALGEBRA Peter M. Higgins
AMERICAN HISTORY Paul S. Boyer
AMERICAN IMMIGRATION
    David A. Gerber
AMERICAN LEGAL HISTORY
    G. Edward White
AMERICAN POLITICAL HISTORY
    Donald Critchlow
AMERICAN POLITICAL PARTIES AND
    ELECTIONS L. Sandy Maisel
AMERICAN POLITICS Richard M. Valelly
THE AMERICAN PRESIDENCY
    Charles O. Jones
THE AMERICAN REVOLUTION
    Robert J. Allison
AMERICAN SLAVERY
    Heather Andrea Williams
THE AMERICAN WEST Stephen Aron
AMERICAN WOMEN'S HISTORY
    Susan Ware
ANAESTHESIA Aidan O'Donnell
ANARCHISM Colin Ward
ANCIENT ASSYRIA Karen Radner
ANCIENT EGYPT Ian Shaw
ANCIENT EGYPTIAN ART AND
    ARCHITECTURE Christina Riggs
ANCIENT GREECE Paul Cartledge
THE ANCIENT NEAR EAST
    Amanda H. Podany
ANCIENT PHILOSOPHY Julia Annas
ANCIENT WARFARE Harry Sidebottom
ANGELS David Albert Jones
ANGLICANISM Mark Chapman
THE ANGLO-SAXON AGE John Blair
THE ANIMAL KINGDOM Peter Holland
ANIMAL RIGHTS David DeGrazia
THE ANTARCTIC Klaus Dodds
ANTISEMITISM Steven Beller
ANXIETY Daniel Freeman and
    Jason Freeman
THE APOCRYPHAL GOSPELS Paul Foster
ARCHAEOLOGY Paul Bahn
ARCHITECTURE Andrew Ballantyne
ARISTOCRACY William Doyle
ARISTOTLE Jonathan Barnes

ART HISTORY Dana Arnold
ART THEORY Cynthia Freeland
ASTROBIOLOGY David C. Catling
ASTROPHYSICS James Binney
ATHEISM Julian Baggini
AUGUSTINE Henry Chadwick
AUSTRALIA Kenneth Morgan
AUTISM Uta Frith
THE AVANT GARDE David Cottington
THE AZTECS David Carrasco
BACTERIA Sebastian G. B. Amyes
BARTHES Jonathan Culler
THE BEATS David Sterritt
BEAUTY Roger Scruton
BESTSELLERS John Sutherland
THE BIBLE John Riches
BIBLICAL ARCHAEOLOGY Eric H. Cline
BIOGRAPHY Hermione Lee
BLACK HOLES Katherine Blundell
THE BLUES Elijah Wald
THE BODY Chris Shilling
THE BOOK OF MORMON Terryl Givens
BORDERS Alexander C. Diener and
    Joshua Hagen
THE BRAIN Michael O'Shea
BRICS Andrew F. Cooper
THE BRITISH CONSTITUTION
    Martin Loughlin
THE BRITISH EMPIRE Ashley Jackson
BRITISH POLITICS Anthony Wright
BUDDHA Michael Carrithers
BUDDHISM Damien Keown
BUDDHIST ETHICS Damien Keown
BYZANTIUM Peter Sarris
CANCER Nicholas James
CAPITALISM James Fulcher
CATHOLICISM Gerald O'Collins
CAUSATION Stephen Mumford and
    Rani Lill Anjum
THE CELL Terence Allen and Graham Cowling
THE CELTS Barry Cunliffe
CHAOS Leonard Smith
CHEMISTRY Peter Atkins
CHILD PSYCHOLOGY Usha Goswami
CHILDREN'S LITERATURE
    Kimberley Reynolds
CHINESE LITERATURE Sabina Knight
CHOICE THEORY Michael Allingham
CHRISTIAN ART Beth Williamson
CHRISTIAN ETHICS D. Stephen Long
CHRISTIANITY Linda Woodhead
CITIZENSHIP Richard Bellamy
CIVIL ENGINEERING David Muir Wood
CLASSICAL LITERATURE William Allan
CLASSICAL MYTHOLOGY Helen Morales
CLASSICS Mary Beard and John Henderson

For more information visit our web site
www.oup.com/vsi/

Aidan O'Donnell

ANAESTHESIA

A Very Short Introduction

OXFORD
UNIVERSITY PRESS

OXFORD
UNIVERSITY PRESS

Great Clarendon Street, Oxford OX2 6DP
United Kingdom

Oxford University Press is a department of the University of Oxford.
It furthers the University's objective of excellence in research, scholarship,
and education by publishing worldwide. Oxford is a registered trade mark of
Oxford University Press in the UK and in certain other countries

© Aidan O'Donnell 2012

The moral rights of the author have been asserted

First Edition published in 2012

British Library Cataloguing in Publication Data
Data available

Library of Congress Cataloging in Publication Data
Data available

ISBN 978-0-19-958454-3

Printed and bound by
CPI Group (UK) Ltd, Croydon, CR0 4YY

Contents

Acknowledgements

This book is dedicated to Hiyam, Ethan, and Maya, for their patience and support while I was writing it.

I have been privileged to practise anaesthesia as a consultant in two fantastic hospitals: St John's Hospital in Livingston, UK, and Waikato Hospital in Hamilton, New Zealand. You have taught, encouraged, inspired, and occasionally terrified me over many years, and in many ways you have shaped the anaesthetist that I have become. You have only yourselves to blame.

My particular thanks to Keith Allman, Vicki Clark, and David Kibblewhite, for their confidence in my ability to write this book. My thanks also to Michael Cooper, Stephen Doyle, Mike Fried, Peter Kempthorne, Andrew Muncaster, Jamie Sleigh, and Iain Wilson for their help with specific questions. I am grateful to the following people for their helpful comments on the manuscript: David Campbell, Margaret Caraher, Gary D'Arcy, Donald Galloway, Alistair Graham, and Mary O'Donnell. Any errors that remain in the text are mine.

I also wish to express my gratitude to Latha Menon and Emma Marchant at Oxford University Press for their help and support during the production of the book, and Alyson Silverwood for her assistance with copyediting.

List of illustrations

Chapter 1
Suspended animation: concepts of anaesthesia

Introduction

A recent study estimated that 234 million surgical procedures requiring anaesthesia are performed worldwide annually. Anaesthesia is the largest hospital specialty in the UK, with over 12,000 practising anaesthetists, yet in many ways it is the most mysterious. Most non-medical people have only the haziest idea of what anaesthesia involves. The media image is unhelpful. Medical dramas, for example, traditionally paint the surgeon as the hero, and the anaesthetist as a panic-stricken subordinate.

When undergoing an operation, the anaesthetic contributes only a tiny part of the overall risk. Yet, in general, people seem to fear the anaesthetic most of all. Many of my patients express real fears, and ask things like 'What happens if I don't go to sleep?', 'What happens if I don't wake up?', 'What happens if I wake up in the middle?', and 'How do you know I am really asleep?'

Anaesthesia is both fascinating and rewarding. What I do every day is to suspend the conscious minds of my patients, so that they can undergo painful, invasive surgical procedures of which they remain entirely unaware. The means by which this is brought about still has a hint of magic for me.

In this book, I give a short account of the historical background of anaesthetic practice, a review of anaesthetic equipment, techniques, and medications, and a discussion of how they work. The risks and side effects of anaesthetics will be covered, and some of the subspecialties of anaesthetic practice will be explored.

Concepts of anaesthesia

Many of us have undergone general anaesthesia ourselves, or we may know someone who has. The concept of general anaesthesia is familiar to us, but it is worth having a closer look at the fundamental aspects.

If you observe an adult male under general anaesthesia, he appears to be asleep. He is lying on his back with his eyes closed, not moving. His breathing is slow and regular. His skin is warm and dry. However, if you were to shout his name, or shake him by the shoulder, he would not wake up. Even if you were to cut into his skin with a scalpel, he would not wake up, move, or show any obvious outward response.

Although we often use the word 'asleep' to describe someone who is anaesthetized (and I usually use this form of words when talking to patients and colleagues), general anaesthesia is not sleep. In physiological terms, the two states are very dissimilar. The term **general anaesthesia** refers to the state of unconsciousness which is deliberately produced by the action of drugs on the patient. **Local anaesthesia** (and its related terms) refers to the numbness produced in a part of the body by deliberate interruption of nerve function; this is typically achieved without affecting consciousness.

What is general anaesthesia?

In the early days of anaesthesia, the mid-19th century, the term *etherization* was used to describe the state produced by the inhalation of ether vapour. However, it soon became clear that chloroform and other agents could produce effectively the same state as ether. Clearly, a patient could not be etherized with chloroform. To try to find one word which sufficed to describe this new state was not easy. Some of the early terms were 'clumsy, and some of them cacophonous', such as *narcotism, sopor, hebetization, apathization, letheonization,* and *stupefaction.* The American neurologist Oliver Wendell Holmes suggested the term *anaesthesia* in 1846 in a letter to William Morton, from the Greek meaning 'without sensation', and this word, together with its adjective *anaesthetic,* caught on rapidly. By the time James Young Simpson was publishing his early results with chloroform in 1847, the term was in common use, although ungainly alternative terms such as *northria* or *metaesthesia* are still occasionally proposed.

The purpose of inhaling ether vapour was so that surgery would be painless, not so that unconsciousness would necessarily be produced. However, unconsciousness and immobility soon came to be considered desirable attributes of anaesthesia. John Snow, the first doctor to specialize in anaesthesia, wrote in 1872: 'Ether contributes other benefits besides…preventing pain. It keeps patients still who otherwise would not be.' For almost a century, lying still was the only reliable sign of adequate anaesthesia. The state of unconsciousness was considered an advantageous relief from the traumatic experience of surgery.

For nearly a century after the introduction of general anaesthesia, it was provided by a single agent in the majority of cases. Usually, this was ether or chloroform; occasionally, a mixture of the two, or switching from one to the other, was used. Since those agents did what everyone thought was required (they kept the patient unconscious and unmoving), no further consideration was needed. However, the introduction of intravenous agents, muscle relaxants, and other adjuncts led to a discussion of the more specific components of general anaesthesia.

In 1926, John Lundy from the Mayo Clinic introduced the term **balanced anaesthesia** to describe using an array of techniques (such as a sedative premedicant to cause sedation together with general anaesthesia using different agents) to obtain best results. In 1950, Gordon Jackson Rees and Cecil Gray from Liverpool proposed a 'triad' of anaesthesia: narcosis (by which they meant 'unconsciousness'), analgesia, and muscle relaxation, which are often represented on a triangular diagram still taught to students. Crucially, one agent was no longer sufficient to produce all of these effects, but by using (for example) halothane for unconsciousness, morphine for analgesia, and tubocurarine for muscle relaxation, safe and reliable operating conditions could be produced. The combination of an anaesthetic agent, an analgesic, and a muscle relaxant is still widely used, but the triad model is out of date. For a better model, a more careful consideration of the components of general anaesthesia is required.

Unconsciousness

A few years ago, an anaesthetist friend dislocated his shoulder playing squash. He went to his local emergency department, where he was given a large dose of the analgesic morphine, and a large dose of the sedative midazolam. His shoulder was then put back into joint. He knows he was awake at the time, and he knows that relocation of the shoulder is an extremely painful procedure, despite the morphine. However, due to the effects of the midazolam, which causes transient memory loss, he cannot remember the pain.

What my friend underwent was not general anaesthesia. However, the question he asked me was whether it is ethical to inflict pain on a patient who does not remember it afterwards, assuming there is no emergency or other urgent reason to do so. After some thought, I replied that I do not think that it is ethical to deliberately inflict pain on a conscious human being at any time, when alternative courses of action are to hand. Whether that person remembers it afterwards is beside the point.

4

General anaesthesia provides unconsciousness, but it is reasonable to look closer at what this actually means.

Among many other functions, the conscious mind is responsible for forming both experiences and memories of those experiences. If only one of those functions were interrupted, the mind might form experiences, such as pain, but not memories, and a situation like my friend's might ensue. However, general anaesthesia temporarily suspends the formation of both experiences (perceptions, awareness) and memories of those experiences.

In addition, general anaesthesia is considered to be a state induced by anaesthetic drugs (the patient cannot make it happen to him- or herself), and one that is reversible, in the sense of not being permanent: if I were to suffer a head injury, I might cease to form experiences or memories, but this is not general anaesthesia.

Muscle relaxation

Another point on the triad model is muscle relaxation. Cutting into muscle, such as the muscle of the abdominal wall, causes a reflex spasm of the muscle itself which makes surgery technically more difficult, and this reaction is only abolished at very deep planes of anaesthesia. Placing a tube in the trachea is also an extremely stimulating procedure, which can only be performed under very deep anaesthesia. Both these problems can be circumvented by the use of drugs to paralyse the muscles. Anaesthesia need therefore only be deep enough to produce unconsciousness, but paralysis sufficient for surgical access or intubation can be readily produced by drugs. The term **muscle relaxants** is used to describe such drugs, which came widely into practice in the 1940s.

However, for many surgical procedures, muscle relaxation is not required. Even without muscle relaxants, a patient under general anaesthesia will not make voluntary movement, even in response to a painful stimulus such as surgery, and immobility to stimulation is one of the easiest objective signs of general anaesthesia.

But unconsciousness and immobility are not the end of the story. Anaesthesia was first introduced as a means of eliminating pain.

What is pain?

All of us have experienced pain, from our earliest experiences as infants teething or with colic.

The International Association for the Study of Pain (IASP) defines pain as 'an unpleasant sensory and emotional experience resulting from a stimulus causing, or likely to cause, tissue damage, or expressed in terms of that damage'. This is a helpful definition, as it incorporates those things which cause pain (actual or potential damage to the body), and the result (an unpleasant sensory experience), as well as the consequences of that result (an unpleasant emotional experience).

The neurophysiology of pain has been extensively studied, and it can be considered to comprise several steps. First, there is the detection of a painful stimulus (**nociception**), which happens by the triggering of specific nerve endings called nociceptors in the skin and other organs. Nociceptors produce electrical signals in pain nerve fibres. These electrical signals are transmitted to the spinal cord by peripheral nerves. The signals may be modified in the spinal cord, but are then transmitted up to the thalamus, a part of the brain which is responsible for integrating sensory signals of all types. From the thalamus, the signals travel to the cortex, the convoluted surface of the brain. At this point, the pain signals are integrated into conscious perception, and it can be stated that pain is being perceived. (Until this point, there were only pain signals.)

However, the process does not end there. The experience of pain triggers powerful emotional consequences, including fear, anger, and anxiety. A reasonable word for the emotional response to pain is 'suffering'. Pain also triggers the formation of memories which remind us to avoid potentially painful experiences in the future. The intensity of pain perception and suffering also depends on the mental state of the subject at the time, and the relationship between pain, memory, and emotion is subtle and complex.

On their journey through the subconscious parts of the brain, pain signals also trigger physiological responses to stress, by activating what is called the sympathetic nervous system to produce adrenaline (the so-called 'fight or flight' response). The effects of adrenaline are responsible for the appearance of someone in pain: pale, sweating, trembling, with a rapid heart rate and breathing. Additionally, a hormonal storm is activated, readying the body to respond to damage and fight infection. This is known as the **stress response**.

Nociception and pain transmission can be demonstrated in very simple animals, such as fruit flies or worms. However, we hesitate to call their experience pain, because we do not consider flies and worms to be conscious in the way that humans are.

To come back to our patient, therefore, it might be reasonable to suppose that someone who is unconscious cannot experience pain or suffering, because experiences require a conscious mind.

In fact, even if our patient does not outwardly respond to a surgical incision, he will show signs of registering the stimulus. His heart rate and blood pressure increase. His breathing becomes deeper and more rapid. The hormonal markers of the stress response can be detected in his bloodstream.

Those responses may be abolished by an analgesic such as morphine, which will counteract all those changes. For this reason, it is routine to use analgesic drugs in addition to

7

anaesthetic ones. But this invites the question: if the patient isn't aware of the pain, why are painkillers necessary?

The hormonal stress response can be shown to be harmful, especially to those who are already ill. For example, the increase in blood coagulability which evolved to reduce blood loss as a result of injury makes the patient more likely to suffer a deep venous thrombosis in the leg veins. The stress response causes breakdown of fats and proteins to mobilize energy stores: the opposite of the healing response required to build new cells and repair tissues. There is therefore a therapeutic imperative to reducing or treating it. Additionally, a patient with good analgesia intraoperatively is likely to wake up more comfortable than one who has not, so there is a humane benefit to good intraoperative analgesia. Typical anaesthetic agents are poor at suppressing the stress response, but analgesics like morphine are very effective. Therefore, the optimal configuration of a general anaesthetic seems to be a general anaesthetic agent to produce unconsciousness, combined with an analgesic to blunt the stress response.

The fridge problem and the formation of memory

As a boy, I remember being puzzled by the question of what happens to the fridge light when the door is closed. Every time I opened the fridge door, no matter how suddenly (to catch it by surprise) or gently (so that the fridge would not notice me), the light was always on. I concluded (wrongly) that the light remained on all the time.

Is there anything which we can measure or detect from outside the fridge, with the door closed, which would tell us if the light were on? It is plain that no light escapes through the door.

Investigation of general anaesthesia poses the same conceptual problem. In this case, the fridge is the patient, and the light is the patient's consciousness. When the door is open, the patient is conscious, and we can clearly see the light, in the form of the patient's interaction with us. When we induce general anaesthesia, we close the door, and we may be left wondering whether the light is somehow still on, however dimly.

One simple solution might simply be to wait until the patient recovers, and ask him what he remembers. The answer is, almost always, that the patient can remember nothing of what happened; in fact, he has no sensation of time having elapsed at all while he was anaesthetized.

By 'remember', I mean explicit memory, which is that memory which can be directly called to mind, such as your home phone number. However, there is also the phenomenon of implicit memory, which is memory which cannot be called directly to mind, but nonetheless informs our choices and actions, without our necessarily being aware of it.

Researchers have studied implicit memory formation under anaesthesia using a variety of methods such as free-association word-pair testing, or hypnosis. Early attempts to reveal implicit memory formation under general anaesthesia seemed disquietingly successful, but were methodologically flawed. To address the issue, a dramatic and compelling study was undertaken by Ben Chortkoff and colleagues in San Francisco. This was essentially a repetition of a 1965 study, but designed to eliminate the flaws in the earlier work by providing both a control group and investigators who were 'blind' to which group the subjects were in. Twenty-one patients were randomized into two groups, anaesthetized, and the following script was played to one of the groups through headphones:

> 'Oh, shit, who turned off the oxygen? Who disconnected the cylinder? Damn it, he's turning blue. God, his lips are blue. Get that thing connected again. You got it? OK. I'm going to give him some more oxygen now.' A 15-second pause followed, during which the lungs were inflated 3 times. 'Ho boy. OK. He looks better now. I think we can continue.'

The control group was played a neutral script, but with the same pause and inflation of the lungs. The following day, each patient was interviewed by a team of three researchers, using questioning and hypnosis to attempt to reveal which script had been heard. The researchers were blind to which script the patients had heard. They were unable to determine which patients had heard the crisis script, and none of the subjects was able to recall the crisis script. Other recent studies designed to investigate implicit memory formation have shown similar results.

Proving that the patient cannot remember things which happened under anaesthesia is not the same as proving that some awareness of those events did not take place at the time. My friend cannot remember having his shoulder relocated, but he believes it was painful at the time. The best evidence we have is that the activity of the brain required to produce consciousness and memory is suppressed very effectively by general anaesthesia.

Arthur Guedel

Arthur Guedel was an American anesthesiologist who was placed in charge of anaesthetic services for the US Army in Vosges, France, during the First World War. The few physician anaesthetists were swamped with cases and could not attend to the thousands of casualties. Guedel trained nurses and orderlies to provide general anaesthesia using ether, and created a wall-chart of the physical signs which took place as an (unpremedicated) patient goes under the influence of ether.

It is plain to any observer that someone who starts to breathe ether starts off wide awake (and, in some cases, fighting and struggling). Then, after a period, the person begins to become drowsy, then very drowsy, then unrousable, then, if administration is continued, the person will eventually die. There is obviously a relationship between dose and effect. Guedel needed to be able to show when the dose was insufficient, satisfactory, or excessive.

Guedel's chart is a masterpiece of clarity and simplicity. It uses observations that are easy and quick to learn (such as the size of the pupils and their response to light, or the pattern of respiration) and require no fancy equipment. Guedel taught his technique to many hundreds of people, and used a motorbike to travel around between field hospitals to supervise and teach his pupils.

Guedel was not the first to describe different stages of anaesthesia. John Snow made an attempt many decades earlier, describing five stages. However, Guedel's stages were easy to differentiate, widely applicable, and very reliable, and became the basis of assessment of anaesthetic depth for the next fifty years.

1. A chart devised by Arthur Guedel as a simple guide to the stages of anaesthesia, using easily identifiable parameters such as breathing and pupillary responses

The first two Guedel stages can helpfully be compared to the effects of alcohol, which are similar in many ways to the effects of general anaesthetic drugs.

Guedel's stage 1 resembles mild intoxication with alcohol. The patient is relaxed and sociable, but otherwise behaviour, memory, speech, and reflexes are more or less normal, although the performance of fine motor tasks (such as driving) is demonstrably impaired. Alcohol, like general anaesthetic drugs, affects different parts of the brain at different rates.

Guedel's stage 2 resembles severe intoxication with alcohol. There are several familiar features of this condition. First, there is a profound impairment of the performance of motor tasks. Second, there is behavioural disinhibition. This is because alcohol suppresses the effect of inhibitory pathways in the brain. This makes drunken people much more likely to act violently, to take foolish risks, or to engage in sexual activity which they later regret. Third, severe intoxication with alcohol predisposes to vomiting, as can be seen demonstrated on city streets after the pubs have closed. Fourth, memory can be impaired. People who drink heavily sometimes cannot remember how they got home the night before, or what their behaviour was like during this time.

Further features of stage 2 correspond to a slight preponderance of the sympathetic nervous system: modest dilation of the pupils (although they will react to light), and a slight increase in heart rate and blood pressure. Some reflexes may be slightly enhanced, because the suppression which normally keeps them in check is lost.

Imagine, then, a patient breathing ether. He is terrified, and in dreadful pain from a gangrenous leg. He knows that if the leg is not amputated, he will die. Reluctantly, he starts to breathe the pungent ether vapour. At first, he is able to cooperate, but then he becomes disinhibited, and his will to cooperate fades. He begins to fight and struggle with the anaesthetist. A few times, he manages to pull the mask away from his face, which slows the onset of the ether. A few strong assistants hold him down, but then he vomits copiously, which causes him to choke and inhale his own gastric fluids.

Guedel's stage 2 is best defined by its most serious problem: disinhibition. Incidentally, fasting the patient before the operation is still routinely practised as a means of attempting to keep the stomach empty. It does not prevent vomiting at the onset of anaesthesia, but it means that the volume in the stomach is as low as possible.

Guedel knew, as many skilled anaesthetists did before him, that stage 2 is the most dangerous stage of anaesthesia. All of the adverse events at induction of anaesthesia occur in stage 2. There are a few additional ones, including coughing, breath-holding, and laryngospasm, a reflex closure of the vocal cords that can cause the patient to die of an obstructed airway.

(It is difficult to get further than stage 2 with alcohol, which is why alcohol is not used as a general anaesthetic agent. Alcohol is not very potent, and must be given orally. Alcohol is also extensively metabolized to poisonous by-products which are responsible for hangover symptoms, but can also be fatal. The lethal dose and the anaesthetic dose of alcohol are therefore quite similar: too similar for it to be contemplated as a sensible choice of agent.)

Despite all these difficulties, it is possible for a gentle anaesthetist to take a cooperative patient through stage 2 and into the safe stage 3. However, during this time, there must be no interruptions, or any loud noises or other stimuli which the patient might consider threatening. For this reason, until recently it was commonplace for anaesthetic rooms to have a sign on the door saying something like 'Do not enter while anaesthetic is in progress'. My surgical colleagues usually ask 'Is it OK to start?' before they insert the scalpel at the beginning of the case. What they are really asking is: 'Is this patient safely through stage 2 and into stage 3?' Although modern agents are much more forgiving than ether, most anaesthetists still ask for quiet at induction.

Guedel's stage 3 is the stage of surgical anaesthesia. This is what is meant by use of the term 'general anaesthesia' today. In stage 3, the patient will lie still, will not move in response to a painful stimulus, and will display no reflex activity at all (for example, the eyes will not react to light) but will have adequate preservation of breathing and heartbeat to remain safely alive. Guedel divided stage 3 into four planes, which are of comparatively little relevance to modern clinical practice.

Guedel recognized that too much ether could kill the patient, and defined stage 4 as the stage of overdosage with anaesthetic. In stage 4, the patient is on their way to death: the pulse becomes impalpable; the breathing becomes very shallow and irregular, and eventually stops altogether. However, at least at first, all is not necessarily lost. Provided that one recognizes what is going on, and stops giving ether, the patient is still likely to recover.

In fact, stage 4 does not come suddenly and unexpectedly. A vigilant anaesthetist watching the pulse and respiration would notice them declining in plenty of time to avert catastrophe.

Depth of anaesthesia

What Guedel did was to formalize, very effectively, a paradigm which everyone had already adopted: the notion that anaesthesia has 'depth'.

The idea that anaesthesia has depth is a compelling one, but also controversial. I believe that the adjectives 'deep' and 'light' as applied to anaesthesia were borrowed from their traditional use in describing natural sleep. Although this makes the metaphor an attractive one because of its seeming familiarity, general anaesthesia is not sleep.

The concept of sleep brings us back to the opening of this chapter, and poses the question: what is the difference between natural sleep and anaesthesia?

Why anaesthesia isn't sleep: looking at brainwaves

The most complete answer comes from studying the electrical activity of the brain, using the technique of electroencephalography (EEG), which was developed in the 1930s and continually refined since. Unfortunately, it is still a somewhat crude method of studying brain activity.

The EEG measures the minute electrical activity of the brain via electrodes placed on the scalp. However, the electrical activity of the brain is not confined to the surface: the brain is a solid organ and the deeper parts of the brain produce activity which may not be discernible on the surface at all, although it is likely that the conscious mind is represented in the cortex. EEG signals are extremely weak, and are measured on the microvolt scale, which makes them prone to interference from other sources of electrical signals, such as the heart or muscles, whose signals are approximately a hundred times more powerful.

The EEG waveform is extremely difficult to interpret. To an untrained observer, it looks like random squiggles. Played through a loudspeaker, it makes a hiss like a radio tuned to static. Trying to work from this signal to deduce what is happening in the brain is extremely difficult. However, certain deductions can be made. Any pathological activity, for example the kind that denotes some types of epilepsy, can usually be identified. And some specific patterns of activity can be recognized; for example, an awake brain produces a fast, random signal known as the beta rhythm, characterized by the presence of activity with a frequency of 16–25 Hz.

Using EEG analysis, sleep is revealed to be a highly structured process. Humans undergo two different kinds of sleep. It is widely known that one of these produces rapid movements of the eyes, and is known as rapid eye movement (REM) sleep, whereas the other is non-REM (NREM) sleep. REM sleep is when the most vivid and evocative dreams occur but accounts for only 15–20% of sleep time. The two forms of sleep occur as part of a pattern lasting about 90 minutes known as a sleep cycle. It is normal to wake transiently between sleep cycles, and have between three and six complete cycles in a night.

Although our perception of sleep is that it is a period of rest and recharging of the inner batteries, 'knitting up the ravell'd sleeve of care', it is clear that sometimes there is considerable cortical activity going on. During REM sleep, for example, the EEG resembles that of the awake individual, with fast, low-amplitude, high-frequency activity.

If we monitor the EEG of someone under general anaesthesia, certain identifiable changes to the signal occur. In general, the frequency spectrum of the signal slows. Some of the features observed seem to resemble those in natural sleep, although the significance of this is not known. Next, the overall power of the signal diminishes. In very deep general anaesthesia, short periods of electrical silence, known as burst suppression, can be observed. Finally, the overall randomness of the signal, its entropy, decreases.

In short, the EEG of someone who is anaesthetized looks completely different from someone who is awake. In contrast to both wakefulness and REM sleep, anaesthesia is characterized by cortical quiescence. As far as we can tell with the EEG, the cortical function needed to create experiences and memories is significantly affected by general anaesthesia, and this is backed up by other experimental evidence.

For investigation of the functioning brain, EEG has been superseded by more effective methods of investigation, such as functional magnetic resonance imaging (fMRI), which can image the activity of the whole brain in real time during specific tasks.

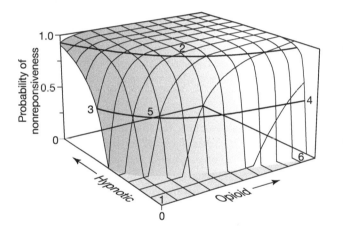

2. **A hypothetical response surface. This graph shows the relationship between opioid (analgesic) and hypnotic (anaesthetic) drug concentrations and the probability of non-responsiveness. Point 1: complete responsiveness. Point 2 and the plateau above: no chance of response. The line at 3 shows the relationship between anaesthetic and responsiveness in the absence of opioid. The line at 4 shows the relationship between anaesthetic and responsiveness in the presence of large doses of opioid. Point 5 shows the area of maximum synergy between opioid and anaesthetic. Point 6 shows that, in the absence of anaesthetic, even very high levels of opioid cannot suppress response. The curved line across the middle of the surface is the 50% isobole: and the curved line across the top of the surface, the 95% isobole. These lines denote a 50% and 95% chance of non-responsiveness respectively**

On the other hand, EEG is non-invasive and compact, and a variety of anaesthetic monitors have been developed which measure a localized EEG signal, typically from the forehead, analyse it mathematically, and distil the result into a single number which can be interpreted by the anaesthetist. For example, 90 to 100 could indicate alertness, 70 to 80 sedation, 30 to 50 general anaesthesia, and zero cortical silence. These systems provide an objective measure of the cortical suppression produced by general anaesthesia.

Depth of anaesthesia is no longer considered to be a linear concept, as defined by Guedel, since it is clear that anaesthesia is not a single process. It is now believed that the two most important components of anaesthesia are unconsciousness and suppression of the stress response. These can be represented on a three-dimensional diagram called a response surface.

The response surface diagram pictured here is hypothetical. A genuine response surface specifies the axes more specifically. For example, it might show the probability of elevation in blood pressure in response to varying concentrations of isoflurane (an anaesthetic) and remifentanil (an analgesic). True response surfaces are determined experimentally: a very time-consuming process. A complete understanding of anaesthetic effects would require response surfaces comparing every possible combination of anaesthetic drugs against every possible surgical stimulus. Although this is a very large task, considerable inroads are currently being made, and it is highly likely that this work will greatly improve our understanding of the processes of general anaesthesia. Ultimately, our understanding will be limited by the complexity of the brain itself, and the evanescent nature of human experience.

Chapter 2
Historical perspective

Inventor and revealer of inhalation anaesthesia:
before whom, in all time, surgery was agony;
by whom, pain in surgery was averted and annulled;
since whom, science has control of pain.

Epitaph of W. T. G. Morton

We live in a world where we consider pain to be, largely, an avoidable experience. Worldwide, the over-the-counter analgesic market was worth over US$30 billion in 2007. For many of us, even a mild headache or sprain has us reaching for the paracetamol (acetaminophen) or the ibuprofen.

Yet, a little over a century and a half ago, things were very different. For most people, especially poor people, pain was more or less a daily experience. There were no readily available analgesics, which meant that pain of all kinds simply had to be endured. Poor nutrition, poor sanitation, overcrowding, and unsafe working conditions created an environment in which problems like rickets, abscesses, and toothache flourished. In the absence of pain relief, childbirth was a dreaded experience for many women.

Occasionally, a person would be suffering so dreadfully from pain that he or she would submit to surgery, without any form of anaesthetic. A limb crushed by the wheel of a cart would, in the absence of antibiotics, quickly turn gangrenous and cause the death of its owner – if not swiftly amputated.

The state of the medical art in the early 19th century was extremely primitive. Medical practice was still largely based on the classical works of Galen and Hippocrates, and harmful practices such as bloodletting were widespread. Nothing was understood about sterility. A surgeon might not trouble to remove his street clothes, or perhaps dress like a butcher, wearing overalls and a leather apron. The patient would require to be restrained by muscular assistants. The best surgeons were the quickest, and could often perform an amputation in less than a minute. Robert Liston of Edinburgh would perform amputations in front of rows of medical students, and begin with the command 'Gentlemen, time me!' and would clasp the bloody knife between his teeth when he needed to use both hands.

In 1811, the writer Frances Burney, known as Fanny Burney, underwent a mastectomy for a tumour that had been causing pain in her breast and arm for over a year. Burney had married a French nobleman, and the operation was carried out in France by Napoleon's surgeon, Dominique Jean Larrey, without pain relief of any kind. Many years later, Burney wrote a poignant letter to her sister describing her experience in detail, and there is perhaps no better account of the patient's experiences:

> Yet – when the dreadful steel was plunged into the breast – cutting through veins – arteries – flesh – nerves – I needed no injunctions not to restrain my cries. I began a scream that lasted unintermittingly during the whole time of the incision – & I almost marvel that it rings not in my Ears still! so excruciating was the agony.
>
> I then felt the Knife tackling against the breast bone – scraping it! – This performed, while I yet remained in utterly speechless torture.
>
> To conclude, the operation, including the treatment & the dressing, lasted 20 minutes! a time, for sufferings so acute, that was hardly

supportable – However, I bore it with all the courage I could exert, & never moved, nor stopt them, nor resisted, nor remonstrated, nor spoke – except once or twice, during the dressings.

Burney survived the operation and lived for a further 29 years.

It is tempting to conceive the surgeons of this period as cold-hearted, bloodthirsty butchers. It is true that some of them had the disaffected air of the showman. Many surgeons, however, were compassionate men who were greatly troubled by the pain they inflicted. Despite her ordeal, Burney noted the traumatized appearance of her surgeon afterwards, and expressed compassion for him.

Before the widespread advent of anaesthesia, there were very few painkilling options available.

Drinking alcohol

Alcohol was commonly given as a means of enhancing the patient's courage prior to surgery, but alcohol has almost no effect on pain perception. Occasionally, a patient was allowed to try to drink himself into a stupor prior to surgery; in most cases, this was probably ineffective.

Opium

Before the birth of modern chemistry in the 19th century, doctors could only turn to the natural world for their remedies: leaves, bark, roots, and so on. Although many treatments were ineffectual at best, and sometimes harmful, some plants do contain powerful alkaloids (drugs derived from plants) which are still in regular use today.

Natural opium is the dried latex of the seed pod of the opium poppy, *Papaver somniferum*. It contains several pain-relieving alkaloids (opiates), of which morphine is probably the most familiar. The properties of opium were known as far back as the Sumerians in the 4th century BC. For many centuries, opium was the only effective pain-relieving substance known. Hippocrates recommended it be used in painful diseases affecting women (but notably did not suggest its use in surgery).

There are, however, several problems with opium. First, the yield of opiates is quite variable. Poppies need warm conditions to produce opiates, which is why Afghanistan is still a very rich source of opium (much of which is now turned into heroin). Poppies thrive in cooler climates, such as northern Europe, but produce almost no opiates. So the strength of opium is unreliable, and therefore the dose cannot be reliably determined.

Second, the means by which opium is administered is unreliable. Many natural opiates, including morphine, are poorly absorbed from the stomach, which means that oral administration is not a particularly effective method. Despite this, laudanum, a solution of opium in alcohol, was very popular as an analgesic. Smoking opium is a very efficient means of delivering opiates, which is why opium dens were so widespread in Victorian times. The invention of the hypodermic needle and syringe in the 1850s greatly improved the efficiency with which opiates (and other drugs) could be administered.

Finally, opium can be addictive. Many doctors and pharmacists, who had ready access to opium, found, after taking it recreationally or experimentally for some time, that they could no longer get by without it.

The nightshades: mandrake, belladonna, and black henbane

The nightshade family, or Solanaceae, includes several species which produce intoxicating alkaloids, of which the most notorious are probably the mandrake, belladonna (the 'deadly nightshade'), and black henbane. The sedative properties of these plants have been known for centuries.

Mandrake, *Mandragora officinalis*, is a highly poisonous plant long associated with both magic and medicine. Its fleshy roots are said to resemble a human figure, but when crushed they yield a powerful cocktail of sedative alkaloids.

Dioscorides, the Greek physician and herbalist, wrote in his *Materia Medica* (c. AD 60):

> The wine of the root of the mandrake shall be given to such as shall be cut or cauterised. They do not apprehend the pain because they are overborne with a dead sleep.

By the 11th century, a potion called dwale was described thus:

> For to make a drink called dwale to make a man to sleep while men carve him.

The author goes on to describe an elaborate recipe containing mandrake, opium, hemlock, and henbane.

Both of these descriptions sound remarkably similar to what we would call a general anaesthetic agent. The pharmacology of the alkaloids involved is consistent with these accounts being quite accurate.

It is not immediately clear why investigation into these techniques was not refined to a higher degree, which might possibly have alleviated a great deal of human suffering over the centuries. I believe the reasons were twofold. First, use of these plants was strongly associated with witchcraft, which would be a strong deterrent to the genuine investigator. Second, as with opium, unreliable yields and

and do hem in a mortar and grynde hem
wel to gedere wiþ youre pyn oile in pyn in
negre in to þe morter a litel at ones and
stire hit to gedere ⁊ so do litel ⁊ litel til hit
be stondyng thik als a oynement ⁊ ley
do hit on a clout and leye an hand brede
a boue þe wounde ouer þe sore til hit be
hol. For to make a drynke þat men
callen dwale to make a man to slepe
whyle men keruen hem. Take thre
sponful of þe galle of barowe swyne
and for a woman of a gylte ⁊ thre
sponful hymlok ius ⁊ thre sponful of
þe wylde nepe and thre sponful of lettu
ce ⁊ thre sponful of pore and thre spon
ful of heulane ⁊ thre sponful of chisil
and medle hem alle to gedere ⁊ boil hem
þan a litel ⁊ do hem in glasen vessel
wel stoppd ⁊ do þer offe thre sponful in
a potel of good wyn ⁊ medle hit wel
to gedere til hit schal be noted and lete
hym þat schal be coruen sitte a ȝen a

3. A late medieval (12th–15th century) manuscript giving a recipe for
dwale, an anaesthetic potion. The recipe is an elaborate concoction of
ingredients, some ineffectual (pig bile, lettuce, vinegar, and bryony
root) and some powerful and dangerous (opium, hemlock, and
henbane). It is likely the author did not know which were which

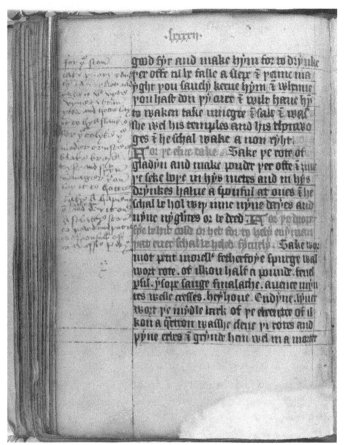

3. Continued

> As nitrous oxide in its extensive operations appears capable of destroying pain, it may probably be used with advantage during surgical operations in which no great effusion of blood takes place.
>
> Humphry Davy

uncertain dosing could easily cause death, which probably made the techniques too dangerous to dabble with.

Mandrake has no place in modern anaesthetic practice, although it adorns the crest of the Association of Anaesthetists of Great Britain and Ireland. However, belladonna has given us atropine, a drug which is still commonly used to increase the heart rate, and henbane provides hyoscine (also called scopolamine), a drug with similar effects. Importantly, neither atropine nor hyoscine is used to cause anaesthesia.

For general anaesthesia to be discovered, certain prerequisites were required. On the one hand, the idea that surgery without pain was achievable had to be accepted as possible. Despite tantalizing clues from history, this idea took a long time to catch on. The few workers who pursued this idea were often openly ridiculed.

On the other, an agent had to be discovered that was potent enough to render a patient suitably unconscious to tolerate surgery, but not so potent that overdose (hence accidental death) was too likely. This agent also needed to be easy to produce, tolerable for the patient, and easy enough for untrained people to administer. The herbal candidates (opium, mandrake) were too unreliable or dangerous. The next reasonable candidate, and every agent since, was provided by the proliferating science of chemistry.

Nitrous oxide

In 1799, the British chemist Humphry Davy was experimenting with different gases, or 'airs', at the Pneumatic Institution for Inhalation Gas Therapy in Bristol, searching for treatments for tuberculosis and other respiratory ailments. In what seems to have been a time-honoured tradition, Davy experimented on himself, by inhaling his new discoveries to judge their effects. Having synthesized some nitrous oxide, he inhaled a few breaths and found it produced a sensation of euphoria. He later found that nitrous oxide had analgesic properties which temporarily relieved dental pain and headache.

Davy recorded in his notebook that nitrous oxide might prove useful in surgery, but thereafter became more interested in its recreational effects, and gave it its common name, 'laughing gas'. No-one seems to have paid any attention to the idea that nitrous oxide might permit painless surgery.

Davy and his co-workers at the Pneumatic Institution invited distinguished visitors to inhale nitrous oxide to experience its pleasurable effects. These demonstrations were soon repeated by students of medicine and chemistry, and then eventually by carnival showmen in both Britain and America. It was to be almost half a century before nitrous oxide was to take its place as a general anaesthetic.

In 1823, English physician Henry Hill Hickman (who invented the term 'suspended animation') performed a series of experiments on animals which were given an atmosphere of carbon dioxide to breathe and became unconscious. Hickman was able to amputate a tail or an ear without any sign of distress, and the animals subsequently recovered. Hickman wrote 'I feel confident that animation in the human subject could be safely suspended by proper means, carefully employed.' Though he wrote to the Royal Society with his results, he was ignored, and died at the age of

30 before he could develop his ideas further. (Carbon dioxide was also a considerably poorer agent than nitrous oxide.)

Anaesthesia and the Victorian era

In the mid-19th century, the impact of the Industrial Revolution, great strides in science, expansion of educational institutions, and the rise of rapid communication and publishing brought wide-ranging cultural changes in their wake for both Europe and North America. The new understanding paved the way for the acceptance of the idea that safe anaesthesia might be achievable. Anaesthesia's time had finally arrived.

In 1844, a New England showman named Gardner Quincy Colton was giving public demonstrations of the entertaining effects of nitrous oxide. One of his volunteers, under the effects of the gas, injured his leg, but seemed to feel no pain. In the audience was Connecticut dentist Horace Wells, who recognized the analgesic potential of nitrous oxide and, after trying it out on himself, successfully adopted it in his dental practice. In 1845, John Collins Warren, a very eminent but sceptical surgeon, invited Wells to demonstrate the anaesthetic effects of nitrous oxide to the medical students of Massachusetts General Hospital, in its new domed operating theatre. He asked for a volunteer from the audience who needed a tooth extracted. A large red-faced man came forward. Wells gave him a few breaths of nitrous oxide from an apparatus he carried. The man's head nodded forward, and Wells then extracted his tooth. The man groaned. The audience erupted in jeers of derision as Wells fled the room. Later, the patient admitted he had felt no pain as his tooth was drawn, but it was too late for Wells, who gave up dentistry in disgrace, and took his own life three years later.

Wells was unfortunate on two counts. Nitrous oxide is not potent enough to be used as a sole agent. A few breaths of pure nitrous oxide will render the patient unconscious, to be sure, but some of this effect is due to oxygen starvation, since nitrous oxide contains no usable oxygen. Next, his patient was large, and large people require more anaesthetic. If Wells had been perhaps a little more careful, and a little less nervous, he might have carried it off.

But the following year, Wells's counterpart William Thomas Green Morton repeated this demonstration in triumph. The setting was the same, and the audience was similar. Once again, the ringmaster was John Collins Warren, whose withering scepticism remained intact. The patient was Gilbert Abbott, a young man with a tumour of his salivary gland. This time, Morton used, not nitrous oxide gas, but ether vapour, which he administered by inhalation from a glass globe of his own design. Ether vapour had been known for some decades to produce similar effects to nitrous oxide, and 'ether frolics' had become commonplace.

Abbott became unconscious from the effects of the ether, and Warren excised his tumour without the slightest sign of discomfort. Astonished, Warren stepped back after the surgery was completed, and remarked to the audience, 'Gentlemen, *this* is no humbug!'

That day, 16 October 1846, became subsequently known as Ether Day, and the operating theatre, which still stands, became known as Ether Dome in its honour. The era of general anaesthesia had begun. Although Morton tried to keep the identity of his agent secret so that he could patent it, the news spread round the developed world as fast as steam and rail could carry it. By December, ether was being used for anaesthesia in Britain and Continental Europe, and the first operations were carried out in Australia in June 1847, and New Zealand in September 1847.

Ether was an excellent, though serendipitous, choice for the first true anaesthetic agent. First, it is easy and cheap to make, by the action of concentrated sulphuric acid on pure alcohol. Second, it is easy to administer, being a liquid which evaporates readily into a

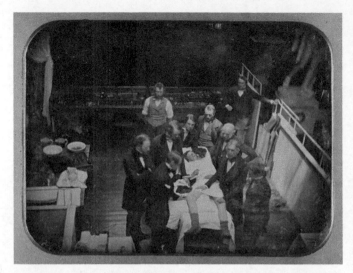

4. A daguerreotype (an early type of photograph) of a re-enactment of the first demonstration of ether anaesthesia at the Massachusetts General Hospital in October 1846. No images were taken on the actual day itself, but a number of re-enactments were arranged for the camera. This one was taken in the spring of 1847. Morton and the original patient are not present but the man with his hands on the patient's legs is John Collins Warren

vapour that can be inhaled. Third, it is potent enough to make the patient unconscious, but comparatively slow in onset, which means it is very difficult to overdose the anaesthetic, especially in a period when surgery was usually over in a few minutes. This means it can be given with comparative safety by novices, and at this time, everyone was a novice.

However, it has clear drawbacks. Ether vapour is pungent and irritant, which makes it very unpleasant to breathe, and provokes coughing and vomiting in the patient. Second, the vapour is explosive, which makes it very hazardous to use in an environment where light and heat were routinely provided by means of open flame.

Every chemist in the developed world started looking through their cupboards for smelly volatile liquids which might be better than ether. The search did not take long.

Chloroform

Edinburgh obstetrician James Young Simpson read the early accounts of ether and was anxious to experiment with anaesthesia himself. A friend, David Waldie, Chemist to the Apothecaries' Company of Liverpool, who was both a chemist and a doctor, suggested to Simpson that another liquid, chloroform, might have some value as an anaesthetic, and provided Simpson a sample. At his Edinburgh home, Simpson passed the bottle around his guests after a dinner party and invited them to inhale it, and the maid came in to find most of the company, including Simpson himself, unconscious around the table.

Convinced he had found the ideal anaesthetic, Simpson began to experiment with chloroform, and applied it to his obstetric practice, where he found it to be useful in alleviating the pain of childbirth. He confidently flooded the medical literature with case reports and descriptions, and was soon regarded as the world authority on chloroform, although his understanding of it was far from complete.

Simpson insisted that administration of chloroform was easy. Liquid chloroform should be dropped onto a loose cone of cloth or even newspaper, held over the patient's nose and mouth.

Chloroform was, in many ways, an excellent replacement for ether. It was a little more difficult to manufacture, but still within the capabilities of a high street chemist. It was non-flammable, more pleasant to inhale, more potent, and quicker in onset than ether. It dominated anaesthetic practice for the next sixty years. But unfortunately, in inexpert hands, it was also deadly.

> Week after week deaths by chloroform are recorded, until at length these events heve become so common that they scarcely attract attention. This cannot and must not be.
>
> *Lancet*, 1854

In spite of Simpson's insistence that chloroform was harmless, John Snow, and later Joseph Thomas Clover, had realized that the haphazard method of administration advocated by Simpson was likely to cause death by overdose. The concentration of chloroform vapour could easily reach dangerous levels.

In 1862, Clover designed an elegant but cumbersome apparatus, in which a specific volume of liquid chloroform was injected into a large airtight bag of known volume, to produce a known, constant concentration of chloroform vapour for inhalation. Clover's apparatus was based on sound scientific principles and worked beautifully – but it was bulky and ungainly, and it failed to catch on.

In addition to the widespread reports of death from overdose, a few reports began to emerge of patients who seemed to die at the very first breath of chloroform. This seemed to occur at any age or state of health, and was reported in patients who were most fearful. This perplexed everyone. A patient could no more die from too little anaesthetic, it was confidently stated, than a person could get drunk on too little whisky.

It took almost a century for this problem to be solved. It is now known that chloroform sensitizes the heart to the actions of adrenaline. Chloroform in a relaxed patient is likely to be safe, but a terrified patient has high levels of adrenaline in the bloodstream. The combination of chloroform and circulating adrenaline predisposes to cardiac arrest, creating the dreadful irony that those patients died who were most fearful of chloroform.

Other chemicals were tried in an effort to find a safe anaesthetic, but all had drawbacks. Combinations were used, such as the 'ACE mixture' of alcohol, chloroform, and ether in specific proportions. Eventually, chloroform was more or less abandoned by the world in the early 20th century – with the exception of Edinburgh – and ether began to achieve predominance once again. But the next big step forward was the change from the inhalational route to the intravenous route.

Barbiturates

Barbituric acid is a cyclical molecule first synthesized by Adolf von Baeyer in 1864, and derives its name from the feast day of St Barbara. Although the bare molecule itself has no direct effect, by modifying its side branches, a wide variety of chemicals (**barbiturates**) can be produced, and nearly all of them have sedative effects on the nervous system. The first to be introduced into medical practice was diethyl barbituric acid (Veronal) in 1903, followed by phenobarbital in 1912.

Barbiturates are versatile and can be administered orally, intravenously, and even rectally. In general, they are very long-acting, and the early barbiturates were used as sedatives for the treatment of insomnia and anxiety. In 1934, thiopental (also called sodium pentothal) was first used in human beings by Ralph Waters, and was found to induce general anaesthesia very rapidly when given by intravenous injection.

Inducing anaesthesia by intravenous injection is substantially quicker than the inhalational method. Inhalational induction may take several minutes, while intravenous induction happens in the time it takes for the blood to travel from the needle to the brain (30 to 60 seconds). The main benefit of this is not convenience or comfort but patient safety. With an intravenous agent, the time spent in Guedel's hazardous stage 2 is substantially reduced.

Anaesthesia can be successfully maintained during the operation by infusing barbiturates, although the elimination of barbiturates is substantially slower than that of ether or chloroform, which means that the patient can take many hours to recover from the anaesthetic. It was soon discovered that the ideal balance is to induce anaesthesia intravenously, but switch to an inhalational agent such as ether or chloroform to keep the patient anaesthetized during the operation. The template of an intravenous induction followed by maintenance with an inhalational agent is still widely used today.

Other intravenous agents followed thiopental, including the barbiturate methohexital, and the agents etomidate in 1971 and propofol in 1977. Meanwhile, advances in organic chemistry produced the first reasonable successors to chloroform and ether. Charles Suckling of ICI introduced halothane in 1951, after methodically testing different fluorinated hydrocarbons. Later, the modified ethers isoflurane, sevoflurane, and desflurane were introduced, and form the mainstay of anaesthetic maintenance today. The term **volatile agents** is used to encompass liquids which evaporate readily and are administered as vapour, and includes these agents as well as ether and chloroform.

The development of anaesthesia was paralleled by advances in other areas of medicine, such as the understanding of germ theory and the adoption of aseptic technique. The subsequent advances in surgical practice as a result have been profound. In addition to the basic drugs and techniques, there is now a large armamentarium of drugs which support the practice of anaesthesia, advanced techniques such as mechanical ventilation, and highly sensitive monitoring equipment. Nevertheless, although highly refined, today's anaesthetic practice has the same fundamental approach to problems which were present a century ago.

Chapter 3
Nuts and bolts

The anesthetist will not be considered a mere satellite of the
surgeon, but recognised as one of a distinct class. There will be an
incentive to men to give their best energies to the perfection of
anesthesia.

Ormond Goldan, 1901

The anaesthetist

The anaesthetist may seem a somewhat obscure figure. In the UK,
public perception of anaesthetists was considered so vague that
in 2001 the Royal College of Anaesthetists declared a National
Anaesthesia Day, an awareness-raising event designed to improve the
public image of anaesthetists, which was repeated twice more.

In the early days of anaesthesia, it was considered by most doctors
that providing anaesthesia was a trivial task which could safely be left
in the hands of students, very junior doctors, and occasionally lay
bystanders. When these novice anaesthetists, through inexperience
or incompetence, killed the patient, which happened far more than is
comfortably acknowledged, this outcome was generally met with a
shrug: the patient was said to 'not take the anaesthetic well'.

A few stubborn pioneers recognized that the safety of anaesthesia
could be greatly improved by careful training and meticulous

attention to technique, coupled with detailed understanding of the underlying physiological processes at work. By devoting themselves to the study of anaesthesia, these men set an example which took the medical profession at large many decades to emulate. The first academic department of anaesthesia in the world was established at the University of Wisconsin in 1933, whose first chair was Ralph Waters. It had taken almost 90 years for it to be recognized that anaesthesia was an academic discipline in its own right.

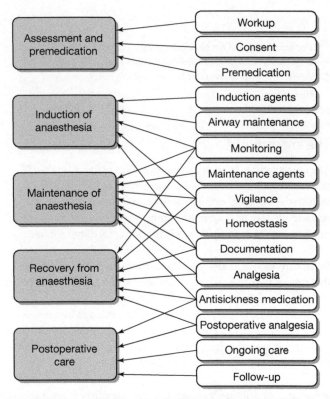

5. **Anaesthesia is a complex process which comprises a blend of many technical and non-technical elements for a satisfactory outcome**

Worldwide, there are many models of anaesthetic care, and it is impossible to describe them all. However, there are some reasonable categorizations.

Doctors

In some countries, the anaesthetist is a doctor who is subsequently trained in anaesthesia. In this model, each anaesthetist is wholly responsible for the care of one patient at a time, from induction, through the procedure, to recovery. This model is the norm in the UK, Australia, South Africa, New Zealand, Japan, China, and Russia.

Nurses

In other countries, the anaesthetist is a nurse who is trained in anaesthesia and who works alongside doctor anaesthetists. The amount of training nurse anaesthetists have is highly variable from one country to another. The amount of autonomy which nurse anaesthetists have is also highly variable, from working under the direct supervision and direction of a doctor to practising completely independently. In 14 states of the US, Certified Registered Nurse Anesthetists (CRNAs) practise without any physician supervision. In the remaining states, nurse anaesthetists practise under the supervision of a doctor. To aid in the differentiation of these roles, the term anesthesiologist, dating back to 1938, may be used to refer to a doctor who is trained in anaesthesia.

One example of this model might be two or three operating rooms working side by side. In each, there is a nurse anaesthetist looking after the patient, and there is one doctor anaesthetist supervising all the nurse anaesthetists, moving from room to room as required. However, there is considerable variability from one country to another.

Anaesthetic nurses are common in the Netherlands, Sweden, Norway, Denmark, Austria, Switzerland, the USA, France, the

Democratic Republic of Congo, Ghana, Tunisia, Cambodia, Indonesia, Taiwan, and Jamaica.

Other

In some countries where trained doctors and nurses are in short supply, anaesthetic care may be provided by a wide variety of individuals. For example, Malawi has one of the lowest numbers of doctors per capita in the world. Anaesthetic care is almost entirely provided by Anaesthetic Clinical Officers, who have no medical training. A similar situation is present in several other countries in sub-Saharan Africa.

It is common for the anaesthetist to be assisted by a technician, whose responsibilities may include preparation and checking of the anaesthetic equipment, fluids, drugs, and other adjuncts to the care of the patient. The training, role, and autonomy of such individuals varies widely from country to country, and there may be considerable overlap between the roles of anaesthetic technicians and anaesthetic nurses.

There is a large number of anaesthetic organizations worldwide, which exist for the ongoing education of anaesthetists. Some cater to subspecialties, such as pain, intensive care, or obstetric anaesthesia. Many of these organizations arrange meetings, at which talks and lectures about anaesthetic practice are given. There are also several medical journals devoted entirely to anaesthesia, in which the latest research and clinical practice is published. As anaesthetic practices continue to evolve, anaesthetists are committed to lifelong learning.

The anaesthetic care pathway

A wide range of procedures may be carried out under anaesthesia of one kind or another. As a general rule, anaesthesia is a bespoke service, which is to say that the specific anaesthetic technique is chosen carefully to match the individual requirements of both patient and surgeon as closely as possible.

On the other hand, there are aspects of anaesthetic care that are present in one form or another for most forms of anaesthesia.

Assessment

Regardless of which kind of anaesthesia is proposed, some form of assessment of the patient must take place beforehand.

A face-to-face discussion with the anaesthetist serves many functions. From the anaesthetist's perspective, it allows the anaesthetist to find out the patient's medical condition. This is done by means of a focused series of questions about the patient's current state of health, past medical history, and medications and allergies, if any. This is known as the **history**. The anaesthetist will ask about any previous anaesthesia and whether any difficulties arose. It is also usual to ask if any blood relatives had any anaesthetic difficulties. There are a very few rare hereditary conditions that make anaesthesia extremely hazardous, and the purpose of these questions is to try to identify someone who may be at increased risk.

This discussion is then often followed by a physical examination of the patient, targeted to any known problem areas, such as the lungs. As part of the examination, it is usual for the anaesthetist to assess the patient's airway by inspecting the mouth, teeth, and neck movement. For general anaesthesia, some form of breathing tube is almost always required, and the airway assessment is designed to show up any potential difficulties in inserting such a tube.

After the history and the physical examination, the anaesthetist may then request specific investigations to further assess the patient's fitness. For healthy patients, or those facing minor procedures, testing may not be required. For patients with very serious disease, or for whom very major surgery is proposed, the testing may be extensive. Blood tests can show up anaemia, possible infection, abnormalities in blood chemistry, and the function of systems such as the kidneys and liver. The electrocardiogram (ECG) shows the electrical activity, but not the structure or function, of the heart. If more detailed assessment of the heart is required, an ultrasound scan of the heart, an echocardiogram, is performed. Pulmonary function can be assessed by measuring the volumes of air the patient can inhale and exhale using maximum effort.

Although these tests can provide very detailed information about the workings of various organ systems, the amount of predictive value they have is limited. A suite of normal results can be reassuring, but is not necessarily predictive of a good perioperative outcome.

The most useful way to estimate the body's physiological reserve is to assess the patient's tolerance for exercise. Exercise is a good model of the surgical stress response. The greater the patient's tolerance for exercise, the better the perioperative outcome is likely to be, though marathon-running is not required. For most patients, the ability to sustain a little light exercise, such as playing a round of golf, or carrying a heavy shopping bag up a flight of stairs, is all that is required.

When I am in doubt about my patient's exercise tolerance, I ask them to accompany me on a short walk up the hospital stairs, which usually clarifies the matter one way or the other. It is possible to put patients on a treadmill and measure their exercise tolerance formally (so-called CPX, cardiopulmonary exercise testing), but this is time-consuming, and is therefore reserved for especially difficult cases.

The next step is called **workup**: to try to improve the patient's condition as much as possible before the operation. For a healthy patient, little or nothing may need to be done. Sometimes, medication may need to be altered to optimize high blood pressure, or blood sugar levels if the patient is diabetic. Stopping smoking is the single most important step any smoker can take to improve future health. For a smoker who is unable to quit, stopping for even a couple of days before the operation improves outcome. Cutting down heavy drinking, losing some excess weight, and starting to take a little exercise (such as a walk every day or a little swimming) can be very beneficial.

On rare occasions, the anaesthetist may discover a health problem which was not previously known, or requires referral to a specialist for treatment before surgery can proceed. In some centres, the business of assessing the patient is partly carried out by a clinic that takes place some weeks ahead of the proposed operation, which allows time for the investigations to be carried out and the patient to be worked up beforehand. In this circumstance, the anaesthetist should still see the patient in person before the operation, even if this is on the day itself.

The second purpose of the pre-operative discussion is to allow the anaesthetist to explain the anaesthetic to the patient. For some operations, only one anaesthetic technique is reasonable. In others, there may be options that can be presented to the patient for discussion. This is an opportunity for the anaesthetist to address any concerns the patient may have about the procedure.

As part of this discussion, it is reasonable for the anaesthetist to mention the risks of the procedure. (The risks of anaesthesia will be discussed in detail in Chapter 8.) Having explained the procedure and its risks, the patient should then be asked to give informed consent to undergo anaesthesia. In some centres, the patient is asked to sign a form giving informed consent to the anaesthetic. This discussion is separate from a similar discussion which the patient will have with the surgeon, covering the details and risks of the surgery itself.

The third purpose of the pre-operative discussion is for a therapeutic relationship to be formed between the anaesthetist and the patient. The patient needs to be able to trust the anaesthetist, and a professional, compassionate, and reassuring manner can go a long way to allaying a patient's anxiety about the anaesthetic.

Premedication

Premedication refers to the administration of some sort of medication before anaesthetic induction to make the process safer or more tolerable for the patient. There are three main indications for premedication: to dry up secretions, to reduce anxiety, and to alter the contents of the stomach.

When anaesthesia was performed by inhalation, the pungency of ether and chloroform caused the patient to produce copious volumes of tears, saliva, and bronchial secretions, which tended to provoke coughing and sometimes vomiting. A medication to reduce secretions is called an antisialogogue. It is no longer routine to administer an antisialogogue, although it may still be called upon for inhalational induction. Atropine (from the deadly nightshade), or its cousin glycopyrronium, may be used for this purpose.

The main, and best-known, indication for a premedicant is to reduce anxiety; a so-called anxiolytic. A calm and relaxed patient not only tolerates anaesthesia better, but is also technically easier to anaesthetize, and is therefore safer. Drugs of the benzodiazepine family, such as diazepam and temazepam, work well when given by mouth, and have two useful effects. First, they are sedative and reduce anxiety. Second, they may interfere with memory formation, which means that the patient may remember less of the procedure.

Anxiolytics are not mandatory, and many patients do not need or want one. Informed consent should be obtained before the patient is given an anxiolytic.

> While it is desirable that there should be no solid matter in the stomach when chloroform is administered, it will be found very salutary to give a cup of tea or beef-tea about two hours previously.
>
> Joseph Lister, 1883

The third indication for premedication is to alter the contents of the stomach. A patient with a full stomach may vomit at induction, or regurgitate stomach contents at any time during the anaesthetic. Stomach contents are highly acidic and contain bacteria and food debris. If they are allowed to enter the lungs (known as **aspiration**), a severe inflammatory reaction can be triggered, which can be fatal.

There are two main things that can be done to reduce this risk. The first is to reduce the volume of stomach contents, which is routinely done by fasting. Prolonged fasting is unpleasant and not helpful. Broadly speaking, the best fasting times are about 6 hours for solid food, 4 hours for clear fluids, and 2 hours for plain water. However, different centres may have different guidelines.

Drugs which encourage the stomach to empty itself, prokinetics, are seldom used. There is no way to ensure that they have been effective.

The second way to reduce the risks of aspiration is to reduce the acidity of the stomach secretions themselves. This can be achieved using antacid drugs such as ranitidine or omeprazole, given some hours in advance of surgery. They work by inhibiting production of gastric acid, but the acidic secretions already in the stomach must be allowed time to pass through naturally.

In emergencies, when surgery is urgent but the patient's stomach is believed to be full, a dose of alkaline solution may be administered, which chemically neutralizes the acid in the stomach. The most widely used solution is sodium citrate, although it has a very unpleasant taste.

Induction

Induction is the term given to the process of putting a patient under general anaesthesia (aiming for Guedel's stage 3). There are two main ways to bring this about. The quickest, and therefore safest, method is to use an intravenous induction agent, such as propofol, thiopental, or etomidate. These are given by slow intravenous injection, with the anaesthetist observing the patient closely to monitor the effects.

However, intravenous induction requires venous access. Some patients, especially children and some needle-phobic adults, refuse intravenous induction, and inhalational induction can be reasonably offered to such patients. Other groups of patients for whom inhalational induction would be reasonable would be patients for whom venous access is impossible (such as post-chemotherapy patients with poor veins) or patients with a very difficult airway, where keeping the patient breathing for as long as possible is desirable.

Inhalational induction is usually carried out using sevoflurane, a distant cousin of ether which has markedly superior properties and is much more tolerable for the patient. However, inhalational induction with sevoflurane takes about three minutes, which is still substantially slower than any intravenous induction. The familiar scene of a shadowy villain holding a chloroform-soaked handkerchief over the struggling damsel's face for about ten seconds, until she succumbs and passes out, is entirely fictional. Sevoflurane is not the quickest in onset of the volatile agents, but it is significantly faster than chloroform.

Maintenance

Maintenance is the term given to the process of keeping the patient under general anaesthesia. Again, there are several ways to bring this about. The two most common methods are to use a volatile agent to maintain anaesthesia, or an intravenous agent. Most induction agents wear off quickly, which means that a technique for maintenance must be commenced immediately after induction has taken place.

Although inhalational agents are comparatively cumbersome to use for induction, they work well for maintenance, and are commonly used for this purpose. Most of the drawbacks of volatile agents disappear when the patient is already anaesthetized. For example, an anaesthetized patient will not object to breathing a pungent vapour. In addition, volatile agents have several advantages for maintenance. First, they are predictable in their effects. Second, they can be conveniently administered in known quantities. Third, the concentration delivered or exhaled by the patient can be easily and reliably measured. Finally, at steady state, the concentration of volatile agent in the patient's expired air is a close reflection of its concentration in the patient's brain. This gives the anaesthetist a reliable way of ensuring that enough anaesthetic is present to ensure the patient remains anaesthetized.

In general, the modern volatile agents have few adverse effects. Most are barely metabolized by the patient. Some agents, such as isoflurane, are cheap to produce, which makes this technique very economical. Inhalational anaesthesia can still be safely delivered using very simple apparatus, and where resources are limited, elaborate equipment is not required.

The second method of maintaining anaesthesia is to use intravenous agents, so-called total intravenous anaesthesia, or TIVA. At the moment, the only agent for which this is possible is the induction agent propofol (often supplemented with the ultra-short-acting opioid remifentanil). For propofol to be used for maintenance, its blood concentration must be very carefully controlled. Unfortunately, it is not possible to monitor the concentration of propofol in blood, so it must be calculated.

Several variables are involved in the calculation. For example, the age, height, weight, and gender of the patient will all affect the propofol concentration in the bloodstream. Next, the metabolic fate of propofol (its pharmacokinetics) must be known. Third, the total dose of propofol already administered must be known. Several algorithms have been developed which take account of all of these variables, and these have been programmed into computerized pumps. The anaesthetist programmes the pump with the details of the patient, and chooses a blood concentration (for some algorithms, a brain concentration can be chosen) for the patient. The pump then administers the propofol in such a way that the calculated target concentration remains constant. This entails giving the propofol rapidly at the beginning of the case, then gradually reducing the infusion rate to keep the target level constant.

TIVA has several advantages. First, propofol wears off more rapidly than a volatile agent. This is especially helpful after prolonged surgery, as the patient will recover consciousness more rapidly after a TIVA anaesthetic than from a volatile anaesthetic. Second, when given in subanaesthetic concentrations, TIVA is a good way of providing reliable sedation. Third, propofol is an effective antiemetic, which reduces the risk of postoperative nausea and vomiting.

However, TIVA also has several drawbacks. The TIVA pump cannot measure the blood concentration of propofol, but only calculate it, and there are several factors which can affect the reliability of the calculation. First, the data which the anaesthetist enters (age, weight, height, gender) must be correct. A mistake in entering data may go unnoticed. Second, and perhaps more importantly, the calculated blood concentration assumes that all of the propofol the pump has delivered has entered the bloodstream. A leaking or disconnected infusion line can allow propofol to be lost onto the floor. If unnoticed by the anaesthetist, this could lead to the true blood concentration falling much lower than the calculated level, putting the patient at risk of awareness. Third, TIVA is currently more expensive than using a volatile agent for maintenance.

In addition to the agent used to maintain anaesthesia, many other drugs may be given as part of maintenance. These can include analgesics, muscle relaxants, antibiotics, intravenous fluids, and medications to improve the heart rate or blood pressure.

During the operation, the anaesthetist remains with the patient at all times. The patient's vital signs are constantly monitored. The anaesthetist ensures that all of the patient's physiological parameters (heart rate, blood pressure, oxygen level, temperature, urine output, position, and many others) are kept as close to normal as possible.

General anaesthesia is somewhat like cookery. Each anaesthetist has a template, a recipe, for how a particular case, such as laparoscopic cholecystectomy or total knee joint replacement, is anaesthetized. The anaesthetist modifies the template based on the requirements of the patient and the surgeon. Each anaesthetist develops their own templates based on their training and experience, and these differ slightly from one anaesthetist to the next. Just as the recipe for the perfect cheesecake may be different for different cooks – but each one tasty – so different anaesthetists may approach the same case in different ways, but with equally satisfactory results.

Recovery

It is a common misperception that general anaesthesia can be reversed by giving an antidote which will rouse an unconscious patient. In fact, no such antidote exists. The anaesthetist stops administering the maintenance agent, and the patient's metabolism removes the agent from the body, allowing consciousness to return.

There is no clear endpoint to a general anaesthetic, and emergence may be a slow process. The patient will emerge from general anaesthesia broadly through Guedel's stages in reverse order. The crucial point is that the patient should be able to maintain their own airway and breathing without assistance. For this to be certain, the patient must demonstrate spontaneous eye-opening or the ability to follow commands. At this point, the airway tube can be withdrawn, and the patient can be left in the care of the recovery nurse.

The recovery nurse monitors the patient's vital signs until the patient is alert, comfortable, and physiologically stable. The patient can then be returned to the ward. Ongoing oxygen, fluid, and analgesia may be administered as required.

Post-recovery

Following prolonged or difficult surgery, the patient may continue to be cared for by the anaesthetist intermittently for a period of several hours or even days. This is usually for ongoing pain relief. Some hospitals have pain teams whose remit is to attend to pain problems following surgery.

It is the responsibility of the anaesthetist to ensure good pain relief following surgery. This may be achieved by giving oral analgesics in many cases. Where the patient is unable to take medication orally, intravenous or even transdermal (applied to the skin for absorption into the bloodstream) analgesia can be used. Other forms of postoperative pain relief include local and regional anaesthetic techniques such as nerve blocks and epidural analgesia.

One of the most popular methods of pain relief is patient-controlled analgesia (PCA). Here, a computerized pump loaded with a reservoir of analgesic (such as morphine or fentanyl) is attached to an intravenous line. The patient has control of the pump via a handheld button. Pressing the button causes the pump to deliver a small dose of the analgesic immediately; thereafter, the pump pauses for a short time (the lockout interval) during which no further presses of the button will result in a delivery. Typically, the pump is programmed to administer no analgesia unless the button is pressed, although a low background infusion rate may be specified. In this way, the patient chooses for themselves how much analgesia is required. Overdose is very unlikely, and the patient can choose the optimal path between analgesic effect and side effects. PCA is very effective, well liked by patients, and can be used even by young children.

Chapter 4
Bells and whistles

The operation room must always be kept in such a condition as to be quickly rendered ready for use in case of emergency... Needles threaded, ligatures cut to proper lengths, sponges of various sizes in bowls, etc. When required it will then only be necessary to light the fire, get a supply of hot and cold water and ice, lay out instruments likely to be required, and have at hand a little wine and brandy.

Henry Burdett, 1880

The anaesthetist has a wide variety of equipment at his or her disposal, most of which is not used outside the specialty. At the core of this armamentarium is the apparatus for maintaining the airway.

The airway

The optimal position of the airway is sometimes poetically described as 'sniffing the morning air': a position where the neck is flexed slightly forwards, but the head is extended slightly backwards. A more familiar description is the position adopted when about to drink from a full pint of beer. In this position, the nose, pharynx, glottis, and trachea are in as straight a line as possible, making the flow of air unobstructed. This position can be maintained easily when the patient is conscious.

In an unconscious patient, muscle tone is lost and the tongue may fall backwards, blocking the airway. This is colloquially (but incorrectly) known as 'swallowing the tongue'. Simple manoeuvres may be employed to relieve this situation: forward displacement of the jaw (**jaw thrust**) pulls the tongue away from the back of the throat and restores the airway. (In the 'recovery position', the head is positioned in such a way that the tongue falls forward, out of the way, but this is unsuitable for most types of surgery.)

The simplest device to apply to an open airway is a face mask. The anaesthetic face mask is designed to sit anatomically over the mouth and nose. It typically has a rigid body surrounded by an inflatable cushion to provide an airtight seal against the skin, and comes in a range of sizes. Formerly made of black rubber, face masks are now made of transparent plastic, which allows the anaesthetist to observe the patient through the mask and to see any vomitus or secretions which may appear. An airtight seal prevents the members of the operating team being exposed to the anaesthetic.

Most anaesthetists can hold a face mask and maintain the airway comfortably with one hand, although it can be difficult in toothless, obese, or bearded individuals. Provided the patient continues to breathe, holding the face mask throughout the operation is a reasonable anaesthetic technique for short procedures, and can be used for much longer if circumstances dictate. In a patient who is not breathing, the anaesthetist may manually ventilate the patient via the face mask.

The application of jaw thrust can be tiring after a while, and a variety of adjuncts exist which make it unnecessary. The oldest and best known is the oropharyngeal airway, invented by Arthur Guedel in 1933 and still bearing his name. The oropharyngeal airway is a short, rigid tube, anatomically contoured to sit in the mouth and hold the soft tissues (palate, tonsils, and uvula) out of the airway as far as the back of the throat (the pharynx). With an oropharyngeal airway in place, jaw thrust is unnecessary, and the anaesthetist may even employ an elastic harness to hold on the face mask, freeing up both hands.

However, although the airway is prevented from obstruction using this technique, the airway is still at risk from secretions or vomitus. An anaesthetized patient will not vomit, but gastric secretions may still trickle passively up the oesophagus if the stomach is full.

To prevent aspiration, the method of choice is to **intubate**: to pass a breathing tube through the vocal cords into the trachea, with an inflatable cuff near the tip. The cuff can then be inflated to make an airtight seal with the wall of the trachea. This creates a very effective seal for ventilation, and also prevents any liquid material from contaminating the lungs. This type of tube is known as an **endotracheal tube** (ET tube). While an oropharyngeal airway *maintains* the airway, an ET tube *protects* the airway, and is still considered the gold standard in airway management.

Two pioneers are responsible for the widespread introduction of the endotracheal tube. In the UK, Sir Ivan Whiteside Magill used uncuffed curved mineralized-rubber ET tubes, which he inserted via the nose and passed blindly into the trachea. They came to be known in the UK as Magill tubes. In the USA, Arthur Guedel demonstrated the safety of cuffed endotracheal intubation in a dramatic fashion. At the beginning of a lecture, his own dog, Airway, was anaesthetized, intubated, and submerged in a glass tank of water. At the end of the lecture, the dog was removed from the water, allowed to recover, and demonstrated that it had suffered no ill effects. This became known as the 'dunked dog' demonstration. (The dog survived many such demonstrations before enjoying a long retirement.)

ET tubes are now usually made of PVC, and come in a wide variety of sizes, to suit all patients. Some tubes are reinforced to resist kinking; others are made of metal to resist laser beams; still others have two channels and two cuffs so that the lungs may be

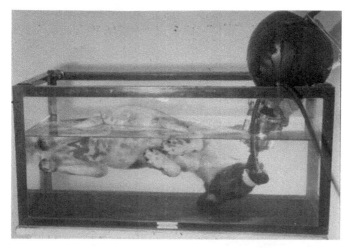

6. The famous 'dunked dog' demonstration was devised and carried out by Arthur Guedel to demonstrate the safety and efficacy of intubating the trachea with a cuffed tube. Guedel's own dog, Airway, was anaesthetized, intubated and submerged in water. The cuff prevented water entering the lungs. The dog survived many such demonstrations before enjoying a long retirement

ventilated individually as required. Very large ET tubes are available for veterinary anaesthesia.

While Magill inserted his tubes blindly through the nose (and some ET tubes are still designed to pass via the nose), it is standard practice to directly visualize the larynx via the mouth and introduce the tube into the larynx under direct vision. The pioneer of the laryngoscope was Sir Robert Reynolds Macintosh, a New Zealander who became Britain's first Professor of Anaesthesia in 1937 (and the second in the world). Macintosh designed an instrument with a curved metal blade, which lifts the tongue and soft tissues out of the way, enabling the anaesthetist to see the larynx and insert the ET tube directly. Although many different styles and techniques of intubation are now used, Macintosh's original blade is still the commonest.

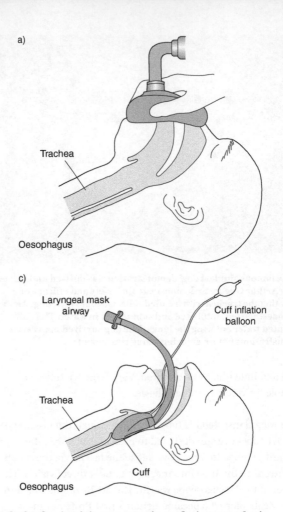

a)

Trachea

Oesophagus

c)

Laryngeal mask
airway

Cuff inflation
balloon

Trachea

Cuff

Oesophagus

7. Methods of maintaining an open airway during anaesthesia
a: The airway is held open by hand, using manoeuvres such as head-tilt
and chin-lift. The face mask must be held on the face by the anaesthetist
c: A laryngeal mask airway sits at the back of the throat above the
larynx. The cuff provides an airtight seal suitable for spontaneous
breathing or gentle mechanical ventilation if required

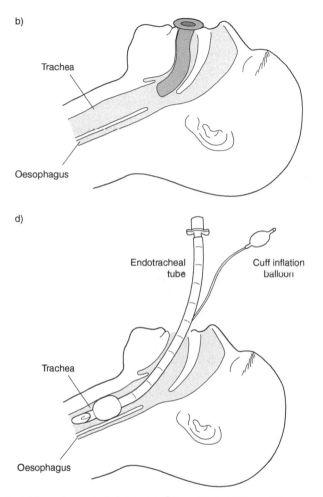

b)

Trachea

Oesophagus

d)

Endotracheal tube

Cuff inflation balloon

Trachea

Oesophagus

b: A rigid oropharyngeal airway may be used to hold the soft tissues out of the way. This is less tiring for the anaesthetist. A face mask is still needed to provide gases
d: An endotracheal tube is inserted through the larynx into the trachea. The cuff makes an airtight seal suitable for full mechanical ventilation. This is the gold standard of airway maintenance but requires skill and deep anaesthesia to be performed

Laryngoscopy and intubation are extremely stimulating. In order to tolerate them, the patient must be deeply anaesthetized, and usually paralysed with a muscle-relaxant drug. This makes the technique less suitable for rapid, short procedures.

The final airway adjunct in common use is a more recent invention designed to circumvent this problem. After years of experimentation with prototypes, UK anaesthetist Archie Brain produced his first commercial **laryngeal mask airway** (LMA) in 1988. The LMA is designed to fit over the larynx (voice box) just as a face mask fits over the face, hence its name. It has a large, soft cuff which, when inflated, covers the larynx tightly, creating a good seal for ventilation. The LMA may be inserted at light planes of anaesthesia, since it does not stimulate the larynx directly, and provides a better seal than a face mask. The LMA was also found to be easy to insert even in patients who were difficult to intubate, although it does not protect the airway. There are now many variants of the LMA, including the intubating LMA, designed to act as a conduit for endotracheal intubation, and the ProSeal LMA, which has an extra channel for the drainage of any gastric fluids which may be regurgitated. The LMA has gone on to become an extremely popular method of maintaining the airway, and it is used for airway maintenance in more than half of all general anaesthetics in the UK (an estimated 1.6 million cases per year).

In the developed world, most airway equipment is designed to be used for a single patient and then discarded, to minimize cross-infection. This is true of face masks, ET tubes, LMAs, and oropharyngeal airways. Disposable laryngoscope blades are also available.

The anaesthetic machine

In the earliest days of anaesthesia, when a bottle of liquid agent and a thick cotton handkerchief were all that was required, the anaesthetist could carry everything around in a leather doctor's

> [Brain] gave us a supply of these [laryngeal] masks and we issued them to our colleagues and said simply 'Poke this down as far as it will go, blow up the cuff, and see how you get on.' And we found to our amazement, in ninety-eight percent of cases, there was absolutely no problem of any sort.
>
> John Nunn, 1998

bag. However, as agents and techniques became more advanced, the equipment became larger, more elaborate, and more cumbersome. Various devices were designed to be worn around the neck of the anaesthetist, keeping everything to hand. However, the death knell of truly portable anaesthetic apparatus was in the early 20th century, with the arrival of compressed gases in cylinders, which were too heavy to be carried.

The anaesthetic machine has evolved to meet a particular set of requirements. Many different types of machine are in use throughout the world, but they all share a common set of features.

First, the machine must have a supply of medical gases. Three medical gases are in common anaesthetic use: oxygen, medical air (purified, dehydrated atmospheric air), and nitrous oxide. The gas supply may come from two sources. First, gas cylinders may be mounted at the rear of the machine. Second, most machines are also connected to a central source of compressed gases which is integrated into the hospital building. Pressurized hoses connect the machine to outlets on the wall of the room. In most hospitals, the cylinders are used only for backup in case the main supply fails.

A cylinder of oxygen may be pressurized to 200 atmospheres (pipeline pressures are lower, at about 4 atmospheres). The highest pressure a patient's lungs can safely tolerate under normal circumstances is about 5% of one atmosphere. A series of regulators within the machine steps the pressure down to safe levels.

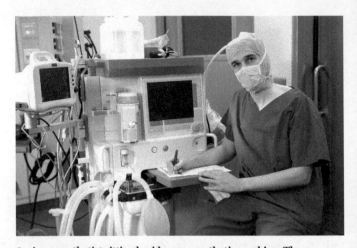

8. An anaesthetist sitting beside an anaesthetic machine. The monitors beside him display readings of the patient's vital signs and the status of the machine and ventilator. The cylindrical object slightly to left of centre is the vaporizer. Beneath this the hoses of the circle breathing attachment can be seen

A bank of flowmeters allows the anaesthetist to choose any gas or combination of gases and deliver a specified flow. The control knob on the oxygen flowmeter is of a different size and texture to the others so that it may be located in complete darkness. With older machines, it was possible to deliver pure nitrous oxide to the patient, which was responsible for some fatalities. All modern machines have a safety interlock to make this impossible.

Next, the machine must have a means of providing a volatile agent. A vaporizer adds a chosen concentration of anaesthetic vapour to the gas mixture passing through the machine. Many machines have two or more different vaporizers mounted.

A vaporizer contains a reservoir of liquid agent, through which the gas mixture from the flowmeters passes. Each vaporizer is calibrated for a specific volatile agent, of which there are only four in common use (halothane, isoflurane, sevoflurane, and desflurane). The desired concentration of vapour is selected by means of a dial. The internal mechanism of the vaporizer produces the desired concentration over a wide range of gas flows. The mixture of anaesthetic gases and vapour is together known as **fresh gas**.

These features together eliminate the practical problems inherent in administration of anaesthetic vapour. A constant fresh gas flow and vapour concentration means that the composition of the patient's inspired gas can be reliably known. The performance of systems which rely on the patient's respiratory efforts to deliver vapour is variable and unpredictable.

Third, the machine must have a breathing attachment, typically a system of lightweight hoses, to deliver the fresh gas to the patient. The breathing attachment may be attached to a **ventilator,** a device for mechanical inflation of the lungs. The patient end of the breathing attachment may be connected to a face mask, LMA, or ET tube.

In its simplest form, the breathing attachment requires two limbs: an inspiratory limb containing fresh gas, and an expiratory limb containing expired gas. A normal adult breath is about 500 millilitres; having a large reservoir bag attached to the inspiratory limb means that the patient can always take a full breath of fresh gas, even if they should breathe in faster than the fresh gas is flowing. The many different designs of simple breathing attachments were arranged by William Mapleson in 1954 into four categories, and he calculated the performance of each using physical principles. They all have the advantage of simplicity of design, but the disadvantage that high fresh gas flows are required to prevent the patient rebreathing (breathing in some expired air), making them very inefficient. A typical adult male breathing quietly at rest inspires about 7 litres per minute of breath (but consumes only 250 millilitres per minute of oxygen). The most efficient Mapleson attachment requires a fresh gas flow of slightly less than 7 litres per minute to prevent rebreathing. In addition, all of the Mapleson attachments behave very differently in spontaneous breathing and mechanical ventilation.

Expired gas differs from fresh gas in several important ways. First, it contains less oxygen and less anaesthetic vapour. Second, it contains about 5% carbon dioxide (CO_2). Third, it is warm and humid. In the early 1920s, Ralph Waters in Wisconsin developed a system to recycle expired air and make it breathable again, using pellets of soda lime, which is predominantly calcium hydroxide. Calcium hydroxide reacts with CO_2 in the expired air to form calcium carbonate, and this reaction traps the CO_2 as well as releasing a little heat and moisture. A little extra oxygen and anaesthetic vapour can then be added to make the expired gas match the fresh gas.

The problem of recycling expired air to make it breathable again is not confined to anaesthesia. Two other groups, astronauts and submariners, face the same difficulties on prolonged missions. One solution is to use calcium hydroxide (or lithium hydroxide), to 'scrub' the CO_2 from the air in the cabin, and a little oxygen may be released in its place.

The circle system is a breathing attachment which incorporates a soda lime absorber. By recycling the expired air, very high efficiency can be obtained, with fresh gas flows approaching only the patient's minimal oxygen requirement (250 millilitres per minute). The greatest advantage of the circle system is economy, but in addition the circle system performs well over a wide range of patients, from infants to very large adults, and performs similarly in both spontaneous breathing and mechanical ventilation. Although much more complex in design, circle systems are now very widely used, and integrated into many anaesthetic machines.

The concentrations of oxygen, carbon dioxide, and anaesthetic vapour can be constantly measured by the machine, which contributes significantly to the safety of anaesthetic delivery. The development of real-time measurement of gases in the 1980s confirmed Mapleson's calculations from 1954.

Positive pressure ventilation

Every anaesthetic machine requires a means of artificially inflating the patient's lungs. A patient who is deeply anaesthetized, or given opioids or a muscle relaxant, may stop breathing. However, a mechanical ventilator is not strictly necessary: the anaesthetist may manually squeeze the reservoir bag to inflate the patient's lungs. This relies on the anaesthetist's constant attention, and the frequency and volume of breaths can be very variable.

Mechanical ventilation is based on the principle of intermittent positive pressure ventilation (IPPV), gas being 'blown' into the patient's lungs from the machine. From its humble beginnings using fireside bellows to inflate the lungs of dissected animals, through its turbulent historical evolution and application to the resuscitation of 'apparently drowned persons', IPPV is now a highly refined technique.

Inflating a patient's lungs is a delicate process. Healthy lung tissue is fragile, and can easily be damaged by overdistension (barotrauma). While healthy lung tissue is light and spongy, and easily inflated, diseased lung tissue may be heavy and waterlogged and difficult to inflate, and therefore may collapse, allowing blood to pass through it without exchanging any gases (this is known as **shunt**). Simply applying higher pressures may not be the answer: this may just overdistend adjacent areas of healthier lung.

The ventilator must therefore provide a series of breaths whose volume and pressure are very closely controlled. Every aspect of a mechanical breath may now be adjusted by the anaesthetist: the volume, the pressure, the frequency, and the ratio of inspiratory time to expiratory time are only the basic factors. One of the commonest means to improve the efficiency of ventilation is to apply a little pressure during expiration, which helps to prevent some parts of the lung from collapsing completely. This is known as positive end-expiratory pressure, or PEEP. Some ventilators can be set to deliver a breath only when they sense the patient attempt to breathe. There are many modes of ventilation which are suitable for different situations. Mechanical ventilation can be continued for long periods of time: patients in intensive care may be ventilated for many days if necessary.

Monitoring

Fourthly, the anaesthetic machine must have a monitor which displays the patient's vital signs during the case. Many countries specify minimum levels of monitoring which must be applied to the patient. These usually include the ECG (measurement of heart rate and rhythm), pulse oximetry (measurement of the oxygen saturation of haemoglobin), and blood pressure measurement (using a cuff applied to the arm), but many monitors are capable of real-time, detailed measurement of the patient's cardiovascular, respiratory, and neurological parameters, as well as body temperature, and composition of the gases in the breathing attachment.

Finally, there are a few other features of the machine. Most machines have a method of removing expired gases from the operating room, and a suction apparatus to remove secretions from the airway. Most machines are built around a chassis mounted on wheels, to make them easy to move around, and have a work surface where equipment can be laid out, and a storage drawer. Modern machines have a large array of safety features: to prevent surges of pressure which might damage the patient or the components of the machine, to prevent the risk of electric shock, to prevent accidental misconnection of cylinders and gases, and so on.

An increasingly common feature of anaesthetic machines is a degree of computerization, to the point where they may be referred to as 'anaesthetic workstations'. Pressures, flows, gas mixtures, and physiological parameters may be measured, displayed, and recorded electronically, and may be linked electronically to centralized data systems within the hospital.

Chapter 5
Anaesthetic drugs and fluids

All anaesthetic drugs are poisons. Remember that in achieving
a state of anaesthesia you intend to poison someone, but not kill
them – so give as little as possible.

Anaesthetics for Medical Students, 1980

Volatile anaesthetic agents

Although ether and chloroform are long superseded, knowledge of
their chemistry provides the key to understanding their successors.

Chloroform is trichloromethane ($CHCl_3$). Recognition of the
structure of chloroform led researchers to explore alternative
agents which are similar. Tetrachloromethane (CCl_4) and
dichloromethane (CH_2Cl_2) are not potent enough. The next logical
step was to add a carbon atom. Ethyl chloride (chloroethane,
C_2H_5Cl), which is quite similar to alcohol, was briefly popular in
the 1920s, but very flammable. Trichloroethylene (C_2HCl_3) has
two carbon atoms united by a double bond, and this agent was
introduced into practice in the 1930s. Unfortunately,
trichloroethylene is chemically unstable, and breaks down easily
into a variety of poisonous by-products.

The 1930s brought rapid development in the chemistry of small
molecules containing chlorine and fluorine atoms, due to their use

as refrigerants. These are now known as CFCs, chlorofluorocarbons. Charles Suckling at ICI in the UK, which had considerable experience with CFCs, sought to find an anaesthetic agent based on CFC chemistry. He came up with halothane (CF_3-CHClBr) in 1951. Halothane is a volatile liquid, a potent anaesthetic, pleasant to inhale, and non-explosive. It dominated anaesthetic practice for 20 years and is still a common agent worldwide.

Anaesthetic ether is diethylether or ethoxyethane (C_2H_5-O-C_2H_5), just one of a large family of ethers. Tweaking the structure of ether to find improvements was also attempted. Early attempts included divinylether (CH2=CH-O-CH=CH2) in 1933, which was just as explosive as ether. As with halothane, adding fluorine to the molecule confers greater chemical stability, making the molecule

Chloroform   Trichloroethylene   Halothane

Ether   Isoflurane

9. A highly simplified illustration of the evolution of modern volatile agents. Chloroform gave rise to trichloroethylene and eventually to halothane. Ether eventually gave rise to isoflurane (as well as sevoflurane and desflurane). However, despite their different origins, halothane and isoflurane have noticeable similarities in structure (shaded area). Many other agents have been omitted from this diagram for simplicity

less flammable. All other current anaesthetic volatile agents are fluorinated ethers. Isoflurane and desflurane are methyl-ethyl ethers (based on the skeleton C-O-C-C), and sevoflurane is a methyl-isopropyl ether (based on the skeleton C-O-C$_3$).

All current volatile agents are colourless liquids that evaporate into a vapour which produces general anaesthesia when inhaled. All are chemically stable, which means they are non-flammable, and not likely to break down or be metabolized to poisonous products. What distinguishes them from each other are their specific properties: potency, speed of onset, and smell.

Potency of an inhalational agent is expressed as MAC, the minimum alveolar concentration required to keep 50% of adults unmoving in response to a standard surgical skin incision. MAC as a concept was introduced by Ted Eger, Giles Merkel, and colleagues in 1963, and has proven to be a very useful way of comparing potencies of different anaesthetic agents. Isoflurane has a MAC value of 1.2%, which means that, at equilibrium (in a steady state), with the concentration of isoflurane in the patient's lungs at 1.2%, then 50% of adults will not move in response to a skin incision. Sevoflurane is less potent, with a MAC of 2%, and desflurane less potent still, with a MAC of 6%. At equilibrium, it is considered that the concentration in the lungs is equivalent to the concentration in the bloodstream, and this in turn is equivalent to the concentration in the brain. Therefore, measurement of volatile agent in the patient's expired breath gives a good approximation to the brain concentration of agent.

Importantly, a patient with 1.0 MAC of any anaesthetic will behave very similarly, regardless of the agent used. MAC values are also additive, so a patient with 0.5 MAC of isoflurane plus 0.5 MAC of sevoflurane can be said to have 1.0 MAC of anaesthetic in total.

1.0 MAC of anaesthetic is sufficient to keep 50% of adults from moving in response to a painful stimulus. Giving more anaesthetic (e.g. 1.2 or 1.3 MAC) will result in far fewer than 50% of adults moving in response to surgery; in other words, MAC correlates with observed depth of anaesthesia.

It has been known for over a century that potency correlates very highly with lipid solubility; that is, the more soluble an agent is in lipid (such as olive oil), the more potent an anaesthetic it is. This is known as the Meyer-Overton correlation, first put forward in 1900.

The next property of volatile agents is speed of onset. Speed of onset is inversely proportional to water solubility. The less soluble in water, the more rapidly an agent will take effect. Desflurane is the least water-soluble of all agents, and has the most rapid onset and offset of all agents, followed by nitrous oxide, sevoflurane, and isoflurane.

The next property of note is pungency. Isoflurane and desflurane are both very pungent, which makes them unsuitable for inhalational induction in most cases. On the other hand, sevoflurane is much less pungent, and has a somewhat fruity smell, which makes it suitable for inhalational induction.

Anaesthetic gases

Nitrous oxide deserves further mention here. Nitrous oxide (N_2O) is a gas which can be compressed into a liquid in the cylinder. Although chemically very different from the agents mentioned above, the same properties can be discussed with respect to nitrous oxide. First, nitrous oxide has very low potency. While the MAC of isoflurane is 1.2%, the MAC of nitrous oxide is 104%, which means that it cannot be reliably used as a sole agent for general anaesthesia (though this can be achieved at hyperbaric pressures). However, since MAC values are additive, it is quite possible to provide, say, 0.5 MAC of nitrous oxide plus 0.5 MAC of isoflurane. The gas mixture would then contain about 52% nitrous oxide, 0.6% isoflurane, and the remainder oxygen.

Nitrous oxide has very low water solubility, which means it is very rapid in both onset and offset. It is also pleasant to inhale, being almost odourless, which makes it quite tolerable for most patients.

Although it is a weak anaesthetic, nitrous oxide is quite a powerful analgesic. Inhalation of a 50:50 mixture of nitrous oxide with oxygen is effective in relieving pain but without being potent enough to cause general anaesthesia. This mixture, known (inaccurately) as 'gas and air', may be offered to women in childbirth. The effects of nitrous oxide on response surfaces (being both an anaesthetic and an analgesic) is complex and incompletely determined. Some obsolete agents such as trichloroethylene and chloroform also have good analgesic properties, but the fluorinated ethers have very little.

The noble gas xenon (Xe) has some of the properties of the ideal inhalational agent. It is odourless, has an exceptionally rapid onset, and, with a MAC of 70%, is potent enough to be given with enough oxygen to use as a sole agent. It also has no adverse environmental impact. Unfortunately, it has some drawbacks. First, it is extremely expensive to produce, being present in only trace amounts in the atmosphere. Second, it will readily diffuse through ordinary anaesthetic hoses, and does not show up on standard gas analysers, so specialized equipment is required to deliver it. Therefore, its use is currently marginal.

Oxygen (O_2) is produced for medical purposes by the fractional distillation of liquid atmospheric air. At ordinary temperatures, oxygen cannot be liquefied, and is therefore stored in cylinders as a compressed gas. At very low temperatures, oxygen may be liquefied and stored in a large tank known as a vacuum-insulated evaporator (VIE). A VIE appears as a tall white cylinder, which may be seen near to hospitals and other facilities. As the liquid oxygen evaporates, heat is drawn from the surroundings, which helps to keep the interior cold.

Medical air is atmospheric air, highly filtered to remove particulate material (such as soot, pollen, and oil droplets), dehydrated to remove moisture, and compressed into cylinders. In addition to being used for anaesthesia, compressed medical air at 7 atmospheres pressure may be used to power surgical tools such as bone drills, without electricity being required.

The anaesthetist may choose an oxygen-air mixture, or an oxygen-nitrous oxide mixture, as the basis for fresh gas for the patient to breathe during anaesthesia. Pure oxygen is seldom used, as it becomes harmful to the lungs following prolonged administration.

Intravenous induction agents

An induction agent is defined as a drug which will induce general anaesthesia in one arm–brain circulation time. There are only three or four in common use.

Thiopental is an ultra-short-acting barbiturate, which was first brought into practice in 1934. It provides rapid, smooth, and stable induction of general anaesthesia, though accumulates noticeably in repeated doses and is cleared from the body only slowly. For this reason, it is unsuitable for use as a maintenance agent, and an alternative agent, such as a volatile, must be used. It also causes a dose-dependent depression of heart rate and blood pressure.

Thiopental is familiar to fans of spy fiction as the 'truth serum' given in subanaesthetic doses to extract information from captured prisoners, although its efficacy here is poor. It is also one of the trio of drugs used (in overdose) to provide lethal injection for judicial execution in the USA.

Etomidate is an imidazole derivative introduced in 1973. Like thiopental, its onset of action is swift and smooth, but etomidate causes very little suppression of the blood pressure. Etomidate is therefore used where maintenance of blood pressure is of concern. However, it has other drawbacks of its own, including the production of twitches and other excitatory phenomena at induction, and the suppression of the synthesis of endogenous steroids by the adrenal glands. This was the cause of a series of fatalities when etomidate was given by infusion as a sedative to patients in intensive care. Although no lasting harm has been proven from a single induction dose, etomidate is unsuitable for maintenance. Etomidate is also likely to cause postoperative nausea and vomiting, and may irritate the veins, causing pain on injection.

Propofol was introduced in 1985, and is probably the most widely used induction agent in the developed world. Propofol is a phenol derivative, and is almost insoluble in water. It is therefore dissolved in soybean oil, which is in turn emulsified with egg phospholipid into a stable oil-in-water emulsion which looks milky white.

Propofol produces rapid and smooth onset of general anaesthesia, with rapid, clear-headed recovery. In addition, propofol is slightly antiemetic, which reduces postoperative nausea and vomiting. Because it is rapidly cleared from the body, it is suitable for maintenance as total intravenous anaesthesia (TIVA). There is a reliable relationship between dose and response with propofol, which means that low doses may be given to provide sedation without general anaesthesia. Large doses will depress the respiratory and cardiovascular systems.

Propofol was introduced into practice at about the same time as Archie Brain's laryngeal mask airway. It was found that propofol suppressed the upper airway reflexes sufficiently for the LMA to be readily inserted in the majority of patients (the same is not true of thiopental). Thus, propofol and the LMA together changed the face of anaesthetic practice.

Alcohol   Propofol   Nitrous oxide

Sevoflurane   Xenon   Thiopental

10. All of these agents possess general anaesthetic properties, despite their very different structures and chemical properties. Nitrous oxide and xenon are gases. Alcohol, propofol and sevoflurane are liquids, while thiopental is a crystalline solid. We now know all of these agents have activity at the $GABA_A$ receptor, although they do not all affect the receptor in identical ways

Ketamine is a very atypical induction agent, introduced in 1965. Ketamine is a derivative of the hallucinogenic drug phencyclidine ('angel dust') and behaves very differently to the other induction agents. Ketamine produces a state of 'dissociative anaesthesia': profound analgesia with only light unconsciousness. In crude terms, most anaesthetic agents suppress consciousness, while ketamine disrupts or scrambles consciousness. Whereas most patients close their eyes and become relaxed and floppy under general anaesthesia, with ketamine the patient's muscle tone may be preserved and the eyes can remain open, and EEG monitors may wrongly conclude the patient is awake.

Unlike other agents, cardiovascular and respiratory systems may be stimulated by ketamine. It is a powerful bronchodilator. It has a slow onset and a long duration of action (10–20 minutes). It can be given by several routes, including oral, rectal, or intramuscular, and it is suitable for use as a sole agent, for example in battlefield anaesthesia. Problems with dysphoria and hallucinations on emergence limit its use.

Mechanism of action of anaesthetic drugs

A very wide variety of agents will produce general anaesthesia. There are two approaches to understanding the action of anaesthetic drugs. First, the molecular basis: what effects do anaesthetic drugs have at the molecular level? Second, the anatomical basis: on which parts of the central nervous system (CNS) do anaesthetic drugs act?

The answer to the first question is complex. Anaesthetic agents probably have effects on many different cellular constituents throughout the organism, and different agents may have subtly different effects from one another.

The predominant molecular basis of general anaesthetic action probably lies with a protein called the $GABA_A$ receptor, a large, cauliflower-like trans-membrane protein with five subunits, found widely in the CNS. The five subunits provide several potential binding sites for general anaesthetic agents and other drugs which may also affect this receptor (such as benzodiazepines and anticonvulsants). The transmitter at this receptor is GABA, γ-amino butyric acid, which is inhibitory (making the post-synaptic cell less likely to fire). Specific binding sites for volatile agents, propofol and etomidate have been identified. When an anaesthetic agent is bound, the activity of the receptor is potentiated, and has a generally inhibitory action. In addition, the $GABA_A$ receptor is found in all the places in the CNS where general anaesthetics might reasonably act.

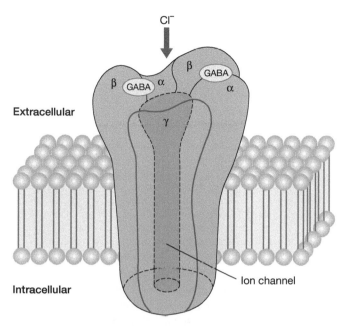

11. A diagram of the GABA$_A$ receptor. The receptor is composed of five subunits which surround an ion channel permeable to chloride ions. GABA, a neurotransmitter chemical, binds to the receptor at two sites, causing the channel to open. General anaesthetic agents and other sedatives such as benzodiazepines, bind to the receptor at other sites, making GABA more effective. The effect of GABA is inhibitory: it makes the neuron less likely to fire. The cumulative effect across the central nervous system leads to general anaesthesia

An additional important role is played by the NMDA receptor, blockade of which produces analgesia. Nitrous oxide, xenon, and ketamine all have effects at this receptor.

The answer to the second question is equally complex. Immobility is produced, not in the brain, but in the spinal cord, by inhalational anaesthetics (but not barbiturates). Two other observable endpoints of anaesthesia, amnesia and unconsciousness, are produced by action on the brain itself. Amnesia probably involves the hippocampus, amygdala, mediotemporal lobe, and possibly other structures; and unconsciousness involves the cerebral cortex, thalamus, and reticular formation.

Where immobility is produced at around 1.0 MAC, amnesia is produced at a much lower dose, typically 0.25 MAC, and unconsciousness at around 0.5 MAC. Therefore, a patient may move in response to a surgical stimulus without either being conscious of the stimulus, or remembering it afterwards.

Muscle-relaxant drugs

Muscle-relaxant drugs are based on curare, the poison used by Amazonian natives to tip their blow-darts. The poison occurs naturally in two vines, *Chondrodendron tomentosum* and *Strychnos toxifera*. The active agent in curare is known as d-tubocurarine. Unravelling the action of curare, which took decades, provided considerable insight into nerve and muscle physiology.

Like curare, muscle relaxants work at the neuromuscular junction, the synapse between the motor nerve and the muscle cell. At the neuromuscular junction, the nerve terminal releases the transmitter acetylcholine, which binds to receptors on the muscle cell to trigger contraction. The action of acetylcholine is rapidly terminated by an enzyme, cholinesterase, which breaks it down in a few milliseconds. This allows very rapid and precise contraction of muscle cells, such as in a pianist performing an arpeggio.

Muscle relaxants paralyse the muscle cell by blocking the acetylcholine receptor and preventing the acetylcholine from binding. Most do this without triggering the muscle cell, and are called non-depolarizing muscle relaxants. Drugs of this family include vecuronium, atracurium, and rocuronium. The other family, of which suxamethonium (succinylcholine) is the commonest example, bind to the receptor and trigger the muscle cell, and are known as depolarizing muscle relaxants. The action of depolarizing agents is accompanied by widespread muscle twitching, known as fasciculation, as they take effect. Muscle relaxants can be easily and conveniently monitored using a device called a peripheral nerve stimulator.

When muscle relaxants were first introduced into practice, some anaesthetists gained the impression that the drugs also produced unconsciousness. To settle this issue, two anaesthetists independently submitted themselves to a large dose of curare, during which they were ventilated through a face mask by a colleague, and subsequently reported that they had been fully conscious throughout. Muscle relaxants also allowed anaesthetists to use less volatile agent than before, creating the potential for one of the most dreaded scenarios in the whole of anaesthesia: the situation where the patient is paralysed, but has not been given enough anaesthetic to remain unconscious during the surgery, and therefore experiences pain. Such a situation is rare, and will be explored more thoroughly in Chapter 8. Pancuronium, a long-acting non-depolarizing agent, is the second drug in the trio given during lethal injection. (Both thiopental and pancuronium are given at much higher doses than would be used clinically; the third drug given is potassium chloride, which induces cardiac arrest.)

On the other hand, muscle relaxation is pharmacologically reversible. For some decades, the mainstay of reversal has been the drug neostigmine, which inhibits the cholinesterase enzyme responsible for terminating the action of acetylcholine at the neuromuscular junction. This results in enormously increased levels of acetylcholine in the synapse, which can displace non-depolarizing agents from the receptors by a process known as competitive antagonism. Unfortunately, acetylcholine is found in many other synapses beside the neuromuscular junction, and neostigmine is associated with major side effects unless a drug such as atropine or glycopyrronium is administered along with it. In the last few years, the drug sugammadex, a ring-shaped carbohydrate molecule known as a cyclodextrin, has been introduced, which binds certain non-depolarizing agents (rocuronium and vecuronium) and inactivates them. It has the advantages of great rapidity of action and very few side effects, but is currently expensive.

Analgesics

Acute pain is the term given to what most of us would recognize as everyday pain: the pain of trapping a finger in a drawer, or twisting an ankle, and is the type of pain which is associated with surgery. The process by which pain is consciously perceived can be broken up conceptually into four stages. Nociception (sometimes called transduction) is the process by which a painful stimulus is detected by a pain-sensing organ, a nociceptor. Nociceptors may be triggered by a variety of threatening stimuli, including mechanical stimuli (such as pinprick), thermal stimuli (such as heat or cold), and chemical stimuli (including inflammatory mediators released by injured tissues). When a nociceptor is triggered, it generates an action potential in a nerve fibre. This action potential carries the pain signal to the spinal cord, and thereafter to the thalamus at the base of the brain. This process is transmission. Finally, pain signals are integrated into consciousness, which is perception.

In 1843, the explorer David Livingstone was mauled in Africa by a lion.

> He caught me by the shoulder, and we both came to the ground together. Growling horribly, he shook me as a terrier does a rat. The shock produced a stupor...It caused a sort of dreaminess, in which there was no sense of pain nor feeling of terror, though I was quite conscious of all that was happening.

Livingstone's experience parallels that of soldiers, who may be seriously injured in the heat of battle, yet experience no pain at the time.

It is clear that the CNS has the ability to modify, and even completely suppress, the perception of pain. This process is known as **modulation**, the best-known theory of which is the gate-control theory, put forward by Ronald Melzack and Patrick Wall in 1965. The theory postulates that pain signals are not carried directly to the brain, but may be modified by other sensory inputs and psychological factors. The key aspect of modulation is that the perception of a painful stimulus and its intensity are not necessarily proportional. A second implication of the theory is that other stimuli can modulate the perception of pain, which is why rubbing an injured limb helps to relieve the pain. There are several sites where modulation may occur; the best studied is the area known as the dorsal horn of the grey matter of the spinal cord.

Anaesthetists have the ability to influence several aspects of this pathway. Local anaesthetic drugs prevent transmission, and general anaesthetic drugs suppress consciousness and thereby prevent perception. It is now accepted that the best method of treating pain is to use several different analgesics, with different modes of action. This technique is known as **multimodal analgesia**. There are two other classes of analgesic which are widely used in anaesthesia.

Drugs which have morphine-like effects are known as **opioids**, which include both natural opiates and synthetic drugs with similar effects. Morphine remains the archetypal opioid, but has been joined by many synthetic or semi-synthetic variants, such as fentanyl, oxycodone, and pethidine (meperidine). Some opioids are weak, and a very few, such as naloxone, oppose the effects of morphine and act as an antidote.

Opioids are very powerful analgesics, and act by inhibiting the conduction of signals in nociceptive pathways. They act on opioid receptors, which are present throughout the CNS, and in some peripheral tissues such as the synovial lining of joints. They have a well-described range of side effects, including nausea and vomiting, respiratory depression, and constipation. They may also cause dependence.

Opioids may be administered in a wide variety of ways to control pain: orally, intravenously, intramuscularly, subcutaneously, by injection into the spinal or epidural space, even transdermally.

The other group of analgesic drugs is the class known as the non-steroidal anti-inflammatory drugs (NSAIDs). NSAIDs work by preventing the synthesis of prostaglandins, inflammatory mediators produced in response to injured tissue. Prostaglandins sensitize nociceptors, which is one reason why an injured part becomes more sensitive to pain afterwards. By inhibiting their synthesis, both inflammation and nociception are reduced.

The original NSAID is acetylsalicylic acid, more widely known as aspirin. Aspirin was first synthesized in Germany at the close of the 19th century and is still one of the most widely used drugs in the world. The next NSAID to be introduced was ibuprofen in 1964, followed by a host of others including diclofenac, naproxen, and indometacin. NSAIDs are very effective in mild to moderate pain, but have well-described side effects, including gastric ulceration, renal toxicity, and a slightly increased risk of bleeding, although they are not associated with dependence.

The most recent group of NSAIDs to be introduced has been the coxib family, which are more selective in their activity than traditional NSAIDs. Coxibs promised the benefits of NSAIDs with a better side-effect profile, and were shown to be very effective analgesics. Unfortunately, they were also shown to substantially increase the risk of heart attack and stroke, and some were withdrawn, leaving only a few, such as parecoxib, still available.

A final analgesic which is often considered with the other NSAIDs is paracetamol, which was first marketed in the 1950s.

Paracetamol's mechanism of action is still uncertain. It does not suppress inflammation, and it shares none of its side effects with the other NSAIDs. It is believed to work in the CNS, and has been shown to be effective in many types of pain.

NSAIDs are most commonly given by mouth, although a few (including paracetamol) may be given by injection or suppository. By combining the use of an opioid, a NSAID, and paracetamol, an effective regime for the treatment of pain can be created.

Intravenous fluids

A wide variety of different intravenous fluids is available, and anaesthetists administer intravenous fluids very commonly. Surgical patients may lose body fluids from a wide range of processes. Bleeding is the most obvious one, but patients may be dehydrated pre-operatively from fluid losses from the bowel produced by vomiting or diarrhoea, or from urine. Pre-operative fasting causes some dehydration by prohibiting drinking. Under general anaesthesia, patients do not usually sweat, but evaporative losses from large areas of exposed tissues may be significant.

The anaesthetist must estimate the patient's fluid status, correct it if necessary, and maintain a good fluid balance intraoperatively. The patient's fluid balance can be estimated using the urine output (if the patient is catheterized), the central venous pressure, and blood tests.

There are four main categories of intravenous fluids: sugary solutions, salty solutions, suspensions of larger molecules called colloids, and blood products.

The commonest sugary solution contains 5% glucose in water. Glucose can exist in two forms, the D form and the L form, of which only one, the D form dextrose, is found in nature. Therefore, the solution is called 5% dextrose in water, sometimes abbreviated to

D5W. The concentration of 5% was chosen because this solution has the same concentration, or tonicity, as blood plasma.

When 5% dextrose is administered, the dextrose is rapidly absorbed by the body's cells, leaving behind only water. It is therefore an effective way to administer water intravenously. (Pure water given intravenously is harmful and causes blood cells to rupture.) It is not, however, a very effective way to give sugar, since there is comparatively little dextrose in a 5% solution. 5% dextrose is therefore an effective maintenance fluid for patients who are fasting prior to surgery, but has few other indications.

There are two commonly used salty solutions. The first is 0.9% sodium chloride, which is sometimes called normal saline. Normal saline has about the same concentration as blood plasma, but has higher levels of both sodium and chloride than blood, which contains many different salts. For this reason, the fluid known as compound sodium lactate was devised by the US paediatrician Alexis Hartmann in 1932 and still bears his name. Hartmann's solution contains sodium, potassium, calcium, chloride, and lactate in levels which mimic those of human blood.

Salt-containing solutions are preferable in the perioperative period, since lost fluid usually contains salts as well as water, and these need to be replaced.

When the patient loses blood, the most important therapeutic step is to maintain the circulating volume. Where blood is not immediately available, salt-containing solutions have some effect. For each volume of blood lost, twice or three times the volume of salt-containing fluid is required for replacement, since salty fluids gradually leak out of the blood vessels into the tissues over time.

However, some fluids are more effective still in the replacement of circulating volume. These fluids contain large molecules which are suspended, rather than dissolved, in water. The large molecules are retained within the bloodstream for longer, since they leak out much more slowly. Such fluids are known as **colloids**. The large molecules may be proteins (such as gelatine) or carbohydrates (such as starches or dextrans). Most colloids also contain some sodium chloride.

Although they can often be very effective, the colloid molecules can cause problems, such as severe allergic reactions (anaphylaxis). They may also interfere with certain blood tests such as the cross-matching of blood products. In themselves, they may slightly interfere with the blood coagulation process, which is highly undesirable in a patient who is already losing a lot of blood. There has been considerable debate in the medical literature about whether colloids are more harmful than beneficial, and this issue remains to be finally resolved.

The final group of intravenous fluids is blood products. Blood products are typically produced from living, non-remunerated human donors, and as such, they are a precious resource. In recent years, there has been considerable change in the use of blood products. For example, the normal haemoglobin level for an adult male is 120 to 140 grams per litre of blood. It has been clearly shown that an otherwise healthy adult can safely tolerate a haemoglobin level of 70. Below 70, a transfusion of blood is likely to do more good than harm. Above a haemoglobin of 70, a transfusion of blood is likely to do more harm than good. This is because the benefit from receiving a transfusion in this circumstance is slight, and may be outweighed by the risks. Risks of receiving a blood transfusion are very low, and include an allergic reaction to the donor blood, or the transmission of a blood-borne infection from the donor.

Donor blood is carefully screened for infectious disease before being fractionated into a variety of products. The red cells contain the haemoglobin which carries oxygen. They are separated, washed, and resuspended in a nutrient fluid before being transfused. A pack of what appears to be blood therefore contains almost no plasma or platelets, but only red cells. The remainder of the blood is a yellow, slightly cloudy fluid called plasma, which contains platelets (tiny, sticky blood cells that promote blood clotting), white cells (which fight infection), blood-clotting proteins, and a variety of proteins of which albumin is the greatest part. Platelets themselves are separated and resuspended for transfusion. White cells are separated off, although transfusion of white cells is uncommon. The remaining plasma is frozen for storage, although it can be further purified into concentrated coagulation factors if appropriate.

Blood products are therefore replaced according to need. Someone who has lost a lot of blood will receive red cells in the first instance. Ongoing bleeding depletes the body's own clotting factors and platelets, and these may be transfused separately as required. Blood coagulation may be tested dynamically using a device called a thromboelastograph, which guides the appropriate use of platelets and clotting factors.

Chapter 6
Local and regional anaesthesia

> A small centipede was rendered completely anaesthetic and
> motionless in the posterior segments of its body, by exposing that
> part alone to the vapour of chloroform for a few minutes. The five
> or six last rings of the centipede, with the suspended and motionless
> feet attached to them, were, for a short time afterwards, dragged
> about in a kind of paraplegic state, by the brisk and lively
> movements of the anterior and unaffected portion of the animal.
>
> James Young Simpson, 1848

This chapter describes the family of techniques which can provide
anaesthesia by interrupting the function of the nerves themselves,
without affecting consciousness.

The nervous system is organized hierarchically. The brain and the
spinal cord together constitute the central nervous system (CNS),
whose function is to integrate the various sensory and other inputs,
process these inputs, and issue commands to the organs of the body.
Surrounding the central nervous system is the peripheral nervous
system (PNS). Peripheral nerves are bundles of nerve fibres whose
sole function is to convey information from the body and its
surroundings to the CNS, and signals from the CNS to the body.

Each peripheral nerve comprises a jumbled mixture of nerve fibres
of all types. Each type of nerve fibre has a specific function. For any

particular nerve, signals may be either heading towards the CNS, known as afferent signals, or heading away from the CNS, known as efferent signals. To avoid the confusion of these similar terms, I shall use **ascending** to describe signals heading to the CNS and **descending** to describe signals heading away from the CNS.

Ascending signals are almost all sensory. There are five sensory modalities (not to be confused with the misleading classical 'five senses'). These are pain, temperature, touch, vibration, and joint-position sense, which is known as proprioception. Touch, vibration, and proprioception travel in the same types of peripheral nerve fibre. Known as A-fibres, these fibres have a large diameter because they have a coating of myelin, a lipid which increases the conduction velocity of the nerve. When they reach the spinal cord, these signals ascend in a part of the spinal cord known as the dorsal columns, on the same side of the body as the signal arose.

Pain and temperature sensation are carried in peripheral nerves in C-fibres. Lacking myelin, these fibres are much smaller in diameter and have a much slower conduction velocity. In the spinal cord, these signals travel in the spino-thalamic tracts, on the opposite side of the body from the signal. Hemisection of the spinal cord, a rare condition known as Brown–Séquard syndrome, leads to loss of touch, vibration, proprioception and motor power on the same side of the body as the lesion, with sparing of pain and temperature sensation. On the opposite side of the body, pain and temperature are lost but touch, vibration, and proprioception and power are spared.

The most familiar of the descending signals are those used to produce muscle movement, so-called motor signals. Motor fibres are type A-fibres. However, other descending signals are below conscious awareness, and regulate the function of internal organs during processes such as breathing, digestion, or childbirth. These signals arise from the autonomic nervous system. (The autonomic nervous system, which also receives ascending signals, is functionally a component of both the central and peripheral nervous systems.)

A nerve cell (neuron) consists of a body (the soma), from which emerge branching processes called dendrites, and a long, thin filament called the axon. The longest axons in the human body are about 1 metre in length. A nerve fibre consists of the axon, plus its myelin sheath, if present, surrounded by a small scaffold of structural material.

Nerve transmission

An individual nerve transmits its signal along the axon by a tiny, self-propagating electrical charge called an action potential. The interior of the axon is rich in potassium ions, whereas the exterior is rich in sodium ions. The interior also carries a weak negative charge (the resting membrane potential). The status quo is maintained by ion pumps on the surface of the axonal membrane, which continually pump sodium out of the axon and potassium in, at the expense of energy. This imbalance of ions and charges creates a zone of potential energy. Opening tiny channels in the membrane allows the sodium and the potassium to switch places, which causes the negative charge to switch to positive for a few milliseconds (depolarization). This positive charge activates adjacent channels on the membrane (voltage-gated ion channels), which allows the zone of depolarization to spread along the axon.

The process is somewhat like knocking over a line of dominoes. As with dominoes, the action potential proceeds at a uniform velocity along the axon. The action potential can be carried in either direction, though in life, neurons only carry action potentials in one direction.

Once the action potential has passed along the axon, the voltage-gated ion channels close, and the ion pumps work rapidly to restore the ion gradient and resting membrane potential for the next action potential.

The action potential is passed from neuron to neuron at the synapse. As the action potential reaches the end of the axon, known as the terminal button, it triggers the release of a chemical, a neurotransmitter. The terminal button lies in close approximation to a dendrite of the next neuron. The dendrite is coated with receptors, which are chemically gated ion channels, which initiate a fresh action potential when the neurotransmitter binds to them.

Other cells besides neurons use action potentials as the basis of cellular signalling. For example, the synchronized contraction of heart muscle is performed using action potentials, and action potentials are transmitted from nerves to skeletal muscle at the neuromuscular junction to initiate movement.

Local anaesthetic drugs are therefore toxic to the heart and brain. In the heart, local anaesthetic drugs interfere with normal contraction, eventually stopping the heart. In the brain, toxicity causes seizures and coma. To avoid toxicity, the total dose is carefully limited and extra care is taken to avoid accidental intravenous injection.

Disrupting nerve transmission

It is comparatively easy to disrupt the function of peripheral nerves. For example, sitting in an awkward position for too long can cause the sensation that one's foot has 'gone to sleep'. This phenomenon is caused by transient compression of one or more of the peripheral nerves which supply the foot. It is harmless and rapidly reversible, though it can be quite unpleasant.

Cold also disrupts peripheral nerve transmission. Fingers and toes can quite easily be rendered numb with cold in wintry conditions.

Dominique Jean Larrey, the same surgeon who performed Fanny Burney's mastectomy, was able to perform painless amputations on wounded soldiers who had lain in the snow for some time, during the Russian campaign of 1812. This effect is known as cryoanaesthesia, and can be produced by deliberately freezing the skin with a mixture of ice and salt, or by evaporation.

Several substances found in nature interfere with nerve conduction by blocking the voltage-gated sodium channels which propagate action potentials. Among these is tetrodotoxin, the venom of the puffer fish, *Takifugu rubripes*, whose flesh is consumed as a delicacy in Japan. However, the most widely known sodium channel blocker in the world is cocaine, the first local anaesthetic.

Cocaine and other local anaesthetics

Cocaine is an alkaloid found in the leaves of the coca plant, *Erythroxylum coca*, which is native to South America. For centuries, the leaves have been chewed by South American people as a mild stimulant and appetite suppressant. Coca was brought back to Europe by the Spanish in the 16th century. Cocaine itself was first isolated by Friedrich Gaedcke in 1855, and an improved purification process was developed by Albert Niemann in 1860. Later, it came to be incorporated into tonic drinks, such as Coca-Cola in 1866, and was available over the counter at Harrods in London until as late as 1916.

In 1884, a Viennese ophthalmologist called Karl Koller, an associate of Sigmund Freud, noted that drops of cocaine solution introduced into the eye produced local anaesthesia sufficient for the patient to tolerate eye surgery. The following year, William Halsted and Richard Hall in New York experimented with injecting cocaine around peripheral nerves, to cause numbness. As a result of their experiments on themselves, Halsted and Hall became addicted to cocaine.

Cocaine has two pharmacological actions. First, it blocks voltage-gated sodium channels in neurons, making it an effective local anaesthetic agent. However, it also acts in the central nervous system, blocking the reuptake of stimulatory neurotransmitters (such as dopamine, serotonin, and noradrenaline) at synapses, thereby enhancing their actions. It is this second action which is responsible for cocaine's stimulant properties, but the accompanying euphoria is responsible for the addictive nature of cocaine. Arthur Conan Doyle described Sherlock Holmes injecting himself with cocaine, to Dr Watson's great disapproval.

For two decades, scientists searched for a drug with the local anaesthetic properties of cocaine, but without its addictive properties. Success came in 1904, to French pharmacologist Ernest Fourneau, who synthesized amylocaine at the Pasteur Institute. Fourneau gave it the trade name Stovaine, after the English translation of his surname. Since then, almost all local anaesthetic drugs have carried the suffix -*caine*. Amylocaine has the same action on nerve fibres as cocaine, but lacks the CNS properties of cocaine. At about the same time, Alfred Einhorn in Germany synthesized procaine, whose trade name is Novocaine. (Simpson had managed to create local anaesthesia in the centipede using chloroform, but failed in his attempts to scale up his experiment to humans, using himself as the subject.)

Amylocaine and its successors are structurally different from cocaine, but all share some common features. Each agent has a ring-shaped 'head', joined by a short linkage to a water-soluble 'tail'. The early agents such as amylocaine and procaine had an ester linkage. This can be broken down in the bloodstream, giving these agents a very short duration of action. In addition, the breakdown products were shown to be associated with a high incidence of allergic reaction. Later agents substituted an amide linkage, which made the molecule much more stable, with improved protein binding and hence a longer duration of action.

The first amide local anaesthetic was lidocaine (lignocaine), synthesized in 1943 by Swedish chemist Nils Löfgren. More recent local anaesthetic drugs include bupivacaine (1963) and ropivacaine (1993).

Topical and local administration

Local anaesthetics are absorbed poorly through intact skin. Therefore, applying them as creams or gels is comparatively slow and ineffective. Despite this, topical preparations are available, such as tetracaine (amethocaine) cream, or lidocaine-prilocaine cream. These creams provide short-term anaesthesia of the skin, for example prior to blood sampling in children.

On the other hand, local anaesthetics are comparatively well absorbed by mucous membranes. For example, benzocaine is an ester local anaesthetic which may be incorporated into throat lozenges to soothe the pain of a sore throat, and lidocaine can be included in gels which treat mouth ulcers or genital itching.

The membranes of the eye are so permeable that eye drops can provide effective local anaesthesia of the cornea and the superficial structures of the eye, for example for removal of a foreign body.

Injecting a local anaesthetic drug into an area of skin will provide numbness of that area for a short while. This technique is suitable for minor surgery such as suturing a wound or removing a mole.

Regional anaesthesia

Halsted and Hall were taking things a step further. By injecting a local anaesthetic drug around a nerve, the function of the entire nerve is interrupted. A peripheral nerve typically supplies a particular area of skin with sensation, and provides motor control to a group of muscles. By blocking the nerve with local anaesthetic, the skin and the deeper structures it supplies will become numb, and the muscles it supplies will become paralysed. This is known as regional anaesthesia. Almost any peripheral nerve can be blocked, with results which depend on its location and function.

Each limb is supplied by several distinct nerves. For reliable surgery on a limb, all must be blocked. For example, the hand is supplied by the radial, median, and ulnar nerves. It is possible, but awkward, to block these nerves individually in the forearm. An alternative technique is to block the nerves much higher up, where they unite in the armpit to form the brachial plexus.

The technique of regional anaesthesia involves inserting a needle near enough to a nerve to deposit the local anaesthetic, but not close enough to injure or transfix the nerve. Early techniques relied on the anatomical landmarks of the patient, but these may vary from individual to individual. Bringing a needle close to a nerve usually causes the sensation of 'pins and needles' (paraesthesia), and this phenomenon can improve accuracy at the expense of increased discomfort from an awake patient. More recently, electronic nerve stimulators have been used to improve accuracy. A nerve-stimulator needle is insulated almost to the tip. A small electric current is passed down the needle, and, as the nerve is approached, the current causes the muscles supplied by the nerve to twitch. This warns the operator when the tip of the needle is near the nerve, but the twitching can be very uncomfortable for an awake patient, and the physical movement of the patient can interfere with accurate needle placement.

With the increased availability of inexpensive portable ultrasound scanners, nerve blocks can now be performed under direct visualization with ultrasound. The operator can see the nerves and observe as the needle approaches. This is also a very good way to avoid injuring other structures, such as large blood vessels, which lie nearby.

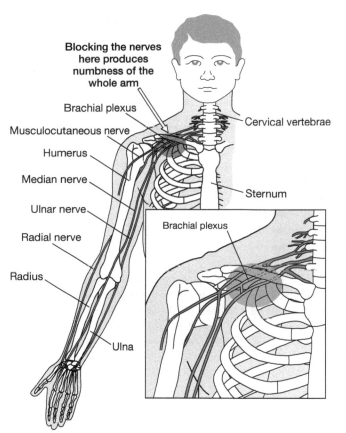

Blocking the nerves here produces numbness of the whole arm

Brachial plexus

Musculocutaneous nerve

Humerus

Median nerve

Ulnar nerve

Radial nerve

Radius

Ulna

Cervical vertebrae

Sternum

Brachial plexus

12. A diagram of a regional nerve block. The arm is supplied by four main nerves which together provide sensory and motor functions. These nerves unite in the armpit to form the brachial plexus. The nerves may be blocked individually in the arm, or one single block of the entire brachial plexus can provide anaesthesia of the entire arm and hand. This block can be performed in several ways

In addition to injecting local anaesthetic around nerves, for long procedures a fine plastic catheter may be introduced alongside the nerves, so that repeated injections, or an infusion of anaesthetic, may be given to prolong the effect.

In expert hands, regional blockade alone may be sufficient for surgery to be performed. For patients who have very precarious health, general anaesthesia may present an unacceptable risk, and a regional technique may allow surgery without putting the patient under general anaesthesia. However, regional blockade is slow in onset, often taking up to 30 minutes to become fully effective, and it is not always completely reliable in preventing all discomfort during surgery.

Therefore, for some types of surgery, regional blockade is performed as an adjunct to general anaesthesia. Typically, the block is placed first, then general anaesthesia is induced. The block can provide pain relief during and after the surgery, and a nerve catheter or infusion can be a very effective way of providing postoperative analgesia.

As an alternative technique of regional anaesthesia, local anaesthetic can be infiltrated intravenously into a limb which is isolated from the circulation by a tight tourniquet. This is called intravenous regional anaesthesia (IVRA), or Bier's block (after August Bier who first described the technique in 1908). The isolation of the limb from its blood supply imposes limits on the duration of the technique, and it tends to be reserved for short procedures.

Spinal anaesthesia

The spinal cord is far more than simply a large nerve. The grey matter of the spinal cord is involved in modification of both ascending and descending signals. Surrounding the grey matter is white matter, which is composed mainly of myelinated axons of ascending and descending neurons. The cord itself is a very delicate structure, coated in a microscopic layer called the pia mater. It is suspended in a clear watery fluid, cerebrospinal fluid (CSF), which circulates around it and the brain, and provides mechanical support. The CSF is enclosed by a fragile membrane, the arachnoid, which in turn is enclosed by a much tougher membrane, the dura mater, or dura. Together, the dura, the arachnoid, and the pia constitute the meninges.

The technique of lumbar puncture, for diagnostic sampling of CSF, was standardized by German surgeon Heinrich Quincke in 1891, although New York neurologist J. Leonard Corning reported two tentative experiments in 1885. Corning produced the first ever spinal anaesthetic in a dog, and what was probably an epidural in a human subject. It is not clear from his description exactly where the tip of his needle lay.

Injection of local anaesthetic directly into the CSF is called spinal anaesthesia. It was August Bier, a German anaesthetist, who took it further, in 1898. As with all the great pioneers, he experimented on himself, in the company of his assistant August Hildebrandt, having first tried it on six patients. This attempt was almost disastrous when Bier lost a great volume of his CSF (and all the cocaine) through a needle which did not connect to the syringe properly. Hildebrandt offered to take his place, and was given 2 millilitres of 1% cocaine solution into his CSF. Bier then tested the technique in a rigorous manner, including pulling Hildebrandt's pubic hair, hard pressure on the testes, sticking a needle into his leg to the bone, and a sharp blow with an iron hammer on the shin. Hildebrandt felt no pain. These experiments were followed by dinner, wine, and cigars.

Both men suffered ill effects from this experiment. Bier was bedbound for over a week and reported terrible headaches whenever he tried to rise (which was due to the loss of his CSF, the so-called dural puncture headache), and Hildebrandt reported vomiting, which was likely to be due to irritation of his meninges by impure anaesthetic, perhaps even contaminated with a little infection.

Bier persevered with spinal anaesthesia for a while, but eventually gave it up due to the toxicity of cocaine. It would require the development of amylocaine and procaine for spinal anaesthesia to regain any popularity.

Spinal anaesthesia provides a dense block of all spinal cord function below the level of the block; a pharmacological disconnection. All sensation is lost, all motor power is lost, and the automatic reflexes controlling blood pressure are lost, which may cause the blood pressure to fall dramatically. The head and upper body remain unaffected, and the patient remains awake, but pain free, during the operation.

The height of the block depends not only on the insertion point, which is usually in the lower lumbar region. Because the anaesthetic solution can spread freely in the CSF, the block height may end up higher or lower than the insertion point. Some anaesthetic solutions for spinal use contain 8% dextrose, making them denser than CSF, so that after injection the position of the patient can be adjusted to use gravity to help position the block height.

There is a limit to how high a spinal block should develop: too high and the muscles that control breathing are paralysed. Higher still and the local anaesthetic drug will affect the brain itself, which causes unconsciousness and sometimes seizures.

Spinal anaesthesia is a routine part of any anaesthetist's skills. It is effective, safe, and quite tolerable for the patient. The local anaesthetic most commonly used is bupivacaine: 2–3 millilitres of 0.5% bupivacaine in the CSF will provide surgical anaesthesia lasting 2 hours or more. Spinal anaesthesia can be performed for almost any procedure on the lower half of the body, including joint replacement, prostate surgery, and Caesarean section.

Epidural analgesia

Surrounding the dura is a potential space containing loose fatty tissue and veins. This is known as the epidural space, or extradural space. In turn, the epidural space is bounded by the bone of the vertebral canal. (In the cranium, there is no epidural space: the dura is enclosed by the bone of the skull.)

Injection of local anaesthetic into the epidural space creates a less dense block than a spinal. The anaesthetic meets the spinal nerves where they cross the epidural space on their path out of the vertebral canal. Axons wrapped in myelin are comparatively resistant to local anaesthetics, which means that unmyelinated axons (those of C-fibres which carry pain signals) are blocked earlier and more completely than myelinated ones. For this reason, a modest dose of local anaesthetic in the epidural space can provide pain relief (analgesia), leaving other nerve function (touch and motor power) spared. A large dose of local anaesthetic will provide a dense block much like a spinal, which is suitable for surgery, although this dose is about ten times greater than the dose required for a spinal.

While injecting through a needle into the epidural space is feasible, the standard technique involves introducing a fine plastic catheter through the needle into the epidural space, and injecting the anaesthetic via the catheter. The catheter can be left in place for up to 72 hours, which means it can be used to provide prolonged analgesia, during and after surgery. Another common indication for epidural analgesia is to provide pain relief during labour and childbirth.

Chapter 7
The different branches of anaesthesia

Ralph Waters was appointed to the first chair of anaesthesia in Madison, Wisconsin, in 1933. In Britain, the Diploma in Anaesthetics, the first academic qualification in anaesthesia, was introduced in 1935, but by the time of the Second World War, only five regular medical officers in the British Army held it.

Since that time, the expansion of anaesthetic techniques has been enormous, and there has been a proliferation of anaesthetists. This expansion in anaesthesia has encompassed two main areas. First, academic research has provided considerable advances in our understanding of physiology in health and disease, as well as the pharmacology of anaesthetic agents. Second, the fields of engineering and physics have contributed greatly to the technology behind the delivery of anaesthesia, and anaesthetic equipment has become highly sophisticated.

These advances in applied anaesthesia have facilitated audacious expansion in surgical techniques. It was prophesied in 1883 that 'the abdomen, the chest and the brain would be forever shut from the intrusion of the wise and humane surgeon'. Now, not only can surgeons freely enter those cavities, but the range of interventions they can perform there is impressive: transplanting organs from one patient to another, or stilling and opening the patient's heart to operate inside it. In 1900, Sir Frederick Treves wrote that anaesthesia 'opened up the craft [of surgery] to many, for in the pre-anaesthetic days the qualities required for success in operating were qualities to be expected only in the few'.

To list all the areas where specialized anaesthetic techniques have an impact on patient care would exceed the scope of this book. However, there are certain specific areas where the expertise of the anaesthetist has particular relevance.

Intensive care

Intensive care medicine (sometimes called critical care medicine) deals with patients who are suffering from sudden failure of one or more organ systems. Patients requiring intensive care are the sickest of all, and require the greatest input in terms of staff, equipment, and interventions, and it is therefore extremely costly. Intensive care is a finite resource, which can sometimes make it hard to decide who should be admitted, and who should not, when space is tight.

In order for intensive care medicine to be established, certain concepts had to be accepted. First, the concept that especially sick patients should be dealt with in units with higher staffing levels than a general ward. This originated in the 'shock tents' of the Second World War, where the most injured soldiers were resuscitated prior to surgery, and later in units set up in European hospitals to treat patients unconscious through poisoning. Second, the introduction of systems that could monitor and record the patient's vital signs continuously, not simply when a nurse was present to take a pulse. Anaesthetic monitoring was ideal for this purpose, especially the monitoring developed for patients following open heart surgery in the 1960s. In tandem with continuous monitoring, more sophisticated blood tests were developed which allowed very precise determination of the patient's condition, including accurate measurement of oxygen and carbon dioxide levels and blood acidity.

The third cornerstone of intensive care was the spread of mechanical ventilation out of the operating room and into the ward. The catalyst for this change was the catastrophic polio epidemics of the 1950s.

In 1952, Copenhagen experienced a severe outbreak of poliomyelitis, a highly contagious viral infection which is usually minor but causes rapid paralysis in a small number of patients. The Blegdams Hospital for Infectious Diseases was inundated with cases of bulbospinal paralysis, patients whose respiratory muscles were affected, as well as the muscles of swallowing. Patients in this unfortunate condition slowly suffocated to death, unable to breathe adequately, nor cough out their own saliva and secretions. The mortality rate was 80%. It was believed that death was caused by viral infection of the brain and that nothing could be done.

The state-of-the-art treatment was to put the patient into a large metal box, with the head protruding from one end through an airtight collar. The pressure inside the box was mechanically cycled upwards and downwards, drawing air in and out through the patient's mouth, mimicking the effect of the diaphragm on respiration. The whole machine was called an iron lung, a misleading term for what was, at best, an iron thorax. It was very difficult to nurse such patients, since access to their bodies was very limited, and very unpleasant for the patients themselves, whose cognitive faculties were unaffected, at least in the early stages of the disease.

The chief physician, Hans Lassen, had too many patients for his few iron lungs. In desperation, he asked an anaesthetist, Bjørn Ibsen, for his ideas. Ibsen realized that the patients were dying of respiratory failure and proposed a technique of manual ventilation of the patient through a tracheostomy, using anaesthetic equipment. After successfully demonstrating this technique, Lassen's misgivings were overcome, and Ibsen's techniques were adopted. The technique was kinder to the patient, who could be nursed in a normal bed, but required constant attention from a carer, to ensure that the airway tube remained open at all times.

There were so many patients that the entire medical and dental student body of Copenhagen was brought in to provide round-the-clock, manual ventilation to the polio victims (mechanical ventilators would have worked just as well, but very few existed at this time). During the epidemic, 1,500 students provided ventilation for 165,000 hours to 800 patients in total. Astonishingly, many patients recovered, and the mortality from bulbospinal paralysis fell to 25%.

It was soon recognized that positive pressure ventilation could be applied to other conditions, such as tetanus, pneumonia, and acute bronchitis. The techniques of mechanical ventilation gradually became more refined and sophisticated. Alongside them came improvements in nutrition, antimicrobial therapy, haemodialysis, diagnostic imaging, detailed monitoring of every organ system, and a wide array of therapeutic drugs and fluids. The understanding of the processes of disease has progressed to the point where specific cells and molecules are now investigated for potential avenues of treatment. Intensive care has now branched out into the specialized treatment of patients with neurological or cardiac problems; burns and trauma; or diseases of the newborn or of childhood. In addition, it is now possible to have ambulances and aircraft fitted out as mobile intensive care units, for the transfer of critically ill patients.

Today's intensive care patient is typically surrounded by machinery and equipment. There is usually a tube of some kind in every orifice. Every possible vital sign is measured and recorded. Every millilitre of fluid administered is charted, along with every millilitre lost. Blood is checked several times daily, and constant adjustments are made to treatment to try to optimize the patient's condition. The patient is constantly attended by at least one nurse with sole responsibility, and a team of doctors reviews the patient's progress several times daily and is always on hand to respond to the slightest deterioration.

Although intensive care can be life-saving, its powers are not limitless. It cannot regenerate worn-out organs, nor reverse years of chronic disease. Those patients do best from intensive care who were previously fit, and are currently suffering from a treatable problem, with the ultimate goal being to restore full function. In most circumstances, the very best which can be hoped from intensive care is for a patient to return to the condition they were in just before they became ill on the current occasion. In UK general intensive care units, around one-third of patients die. Other units and countries may have different figures, though this does not necessarily reflect better or poorer care; a region with more intensive care beds per head of population can afford to admit patients who are slightly less sick, and therefore less likely to die, and their mortality figures may be lower.

Pain medicine

To say that anaesthetists treat pain seems almost absurdly simplistic, but the understanding and treatment of pain has reached a very high level of sophistication. In addition to common types of acute pain, such as that caused by injury or surgery, there are some unusual types of pain which are resistant to normal painkilling techniques. This wide range of pain disorders is encompassed under the term **chronic pain**.

The terms 'acute pain' and 'chronic pain' are intended to describe patterns of pain; they do not convey information about the severity of the pain, although their colloquial use in this regard may be misleading ('the pain in my back was something chronic').

Acute pain, such as surgical pain, can usually be expected to diminish with time. Wounds heal, inflammation subsides, and pain resolves. Chronic pain, on the other hand, is notable for its persistence over long periods of time. During this time, it may evolve and even get worse. Chronic pain may result from prolonged acute pain, such as that of a non-healing ulcer, or from an abnormality in the nervous system itself, which disrupts the normal mechanisms of nociception, transmission, and modulation.

One example of chronic pain is the pain caused by a prolapsed intervertebral disc (a 'slipped disc'), which can press on a spinal nerve as it emerges between the vertebrae. The pain fibres in the compressed nerve are triggered, causing the sensation of pain in the leg and foot, although the leg is not the site of the problem but the nerve itself. Pain caused by nerve damage is known as **neuropathic pain**. Neuropathic pain may have an unfamiliar, strange character; it may worsen unprovoked, or be elicited by otherwise innocent stimuli, such as air blowing over the skin, and it is frustratingly unresponsive to traditional analgesics such as opioids and NSAIDS.

Chronic pain is associated with demonstrable changes in cellular connections and signalling in the nervous system itself, known as **central wind-up**, which may paradoxically intensify the perception of pain with time. In addition, the presence of unrelenting pain may have a significant impact on the sufferer's quality of life: appetite, sleep, and relationships may be adversely affected. In turn, the normal ups and downs of a person's life can greatly affect their perception of, and ability to cope with, their pain. One of the challenging aspects of pain medicine is that pain is an entirely subjective experience: no scan or test will objectively reveal pain, which means that a therapeutic relationship built on trust is a fundamental component of pain medicine.

The recognition of pain itself as a disease, rather than merely a manifestation of another pathology, was championed by John

Bonica, an Italian-born New York anesthesiologist who was extensively involved in the treatment of chronic pain in soldiers injured in the Second World War. Bonica realized that the diagnosis and treatment of patients with chronic pain was optimized by the inclusion of specialists from several disciplines, such as neurosurgery, psychology, and physiotherapy. In 1961, he set up the first multidisciplinary pain clinic, in Tacoma, Washington, and this model forms the basis for chronic pain management worldwide. Bonica later went on to found the International Association for the Study of Pain in 1973. IASP defines chronic pain as 'pain without apparent biological value that has persisted beyond the normal tissue healing time, usually taken to be 3 months'.

The treatments for chronic pain come from several disciplines. Traditional analgesics may have only a marginal effect, but many other drugs have been found to be useful, including the anticonvulsants carbamazepine and gabapentin, the antidepressant amitriptyline, the hormone calcitonin, and the fiery extract of chilli pepper, capsaicin. Other interventions include nerve blocks, and even implantable devices such as spinal cord stimulators. These are supported by psychological treatments such as cognitive behavioural therapy.

Obstetrics

Chloroform is a decoy of Satan, apparently offering itself to bless women, but in the end it will harden society and rob God of the deep earnest cries which arise in time of trouble for help.

Anonymous clergyman in a letter to Simpson

Having been brought up to think it remarkable that after centuries of agony and death in childbirth women had finally been offered anaesthetics, it takes me some time to come around to the notion of natural birth.

Rachel Cusk

Pain relief in childbirth is a well-known aspect of modern anaesthetic care, and has aroused controversy since its beginnings.

James Young Simpson, an obstetrician, applied first ether and then chloroform to women in labour. He was so impressed with the results that he became an outspoken advocate of its use. Though his views met with popular approval, other obstetricians and the occasional clergyman opposed him, both groups insisting that pain in childbirth was not only natural but essential.

Simpson robustly defended his position, but what settled the matter was Queen Victoria, who insisted on chloroform at the birth of her eighth child, Prince Leopold, in 1853, and again at the birth of Princess Beatrice in 1857. The anaesthetist in each case was John Snow. Victoria wrote: 'Dr. Snow gave that blessed chloroform and the effect was soothing, quieting and delightful beyond measure.' The royal seal of approval effectively silenced the objectors, and Snow's technique became known as *anaesthésie à la reine.*

Snow's technique was not general anaesthesia. He was aiming for two things: partial loss of consciousness, and analgesia. He achieved this with light and repeated doses of chloroform throughout labour. Later, the seductively named technique of 'twilight sleep' (*Dammerschlaf*) was introduced in Austria in 1903. It used a combination of injected morphine and hyoscine (scopolamine) to achieve the same ends, and was popular for some decades.

But some of Simpson's critics were correct: it is now known that general anaesthetic agents (including current volatile agents) inhibit uterine contractions, making them less frequent and less powerful, and hence prolong labour. In addition, powerful analgesics like morphine cross the placenta and affect the baby, making it sleepy and less inclined to breathe at delivery.

Today, there are three proven methods of pain relief in labour. First, a mixture of nitrous oxide with oxygen may be breathed by the mother as required. Nitrous oxide has a rapid onset and offset (within a minute or so), affects consciousness only moderately, and is an effective analgesic. The oxygen ensures that both mother and baby receive plenty of oxygen during its use, and therefore the technique is very safe.

Second, an opioid may be given by injection. Drugs used in this way include morphine, diamorphine, and pethidine. The ultra-short-acting remifentanil can be given by a patient-controlled pump, and acts for a little longer than one uterine contraction, but requires regular contractions and a bit of practice to work reliably. Opioids are used cautiously because of their effects on the baby.

The third, and most effective, method of pain relief is to inject local anaesthetic drugs through an epidural catheter. This has no effect on the patient's consciousness, and has no direct adverse effects on the baby. Modern anaesthetic regimes have minimal impact on movement and other sensations beside pain, giving rise to the 'walking epidural' in which the mother retains mobility and the muscular power to push.

There are other ways to feel better in labour besides calling the anaesthetist. The presence of a partner, a supportive midwife, and labouring in pleasant, non-threatening surroundings can be helpful, as can education and preparation for the experience. Some women do not require analgesia; others choose to decline it. However, for those women who ask for analgesia, I believe they are entitled to have it provided promptly and to the highest possible standard by a trained practitioner.

For Caesarean section, in most cases spinal anaesthesia is the technique of choice (an epidural can be topped up to achieve almost the same effect). This allows the mother to remain awake and see her baby immediately after delivery. Spinal anaesthesia is also slightly safer than general anaesthesia in pregnant women, who have physiological changes which make general anaesthesia riskier and more difficult, although it is employed when necessary, such as in emergencies.

Epidural anaesthesia is associated with a longer labour and a higher risk of instrumental delivery or Caesarean. Critics argue that this means that epidurals prolong labour and inhibit natural delivery, but correlation does not prove causation. An equally valid view is that a subset of women in labour have a pre-existing problem which, for them, will make labour longer and more difficult. These women are therefore more likely to request epidural analgesia, but this does not make the epidural the cause of the longer labour or the difficult delivery.

Paediatric anaesthesia

> … a protracted and sanguine battle between surgeon and
> anaesthetist with the poor unfortunate baby as the battlefield.
>
> A description of early paediatric anaesthesia by Philip Ayre

James Young Simpson published an early case report of chloroform in 1847, in which 'a boy, four or five years old, with necrosis of one of the bones of the forearm' was anaesthetized with chloroform:

> A deep incision was now made down to the diseased bone; and by the use of the forceps, nearly the whole of the radius, in the state of sequestrum [dead bone], was extracted.' Half an hour after the operation, he was noted to have 'a clear merry eye and placid expression of countenance. On being shown his wounded arm, he looked much surprised, but neither cried nor otherwise expressed the slightest alarm.

This is an extraordinary account. There is no mention of the child receiving any sort of analgesia, yet he seemed to be pain-free after a serious and quite mutilating operation. I wonder whether Simpson was sugaring his description somewhat. In any case, Simpson, through no fault of his own, was committing the error of considering children as if they were small adults.

In fact, the physiology of children is quite distinct from that of adults, and that of very young children, such as newborn and even preterm babies, is very different indeed. This means that they react differently to anaesthetic drugs compared to adults; for example, the newborn's immature liver cannot metabolize some drugs as quickly as would be expected. Their rapid metabolism and lack of physiological reserve means that catastrophe is always much closer when anaesthetizing an infant than an adult.

In addition, everything about children is not simply smaller, but also differently proportioned. Many techniques, including access to the airway or the circulation, are more fiddly than in adults. This has necessitated redesigning almost everything for use in paediatric anaesthesia (such as airway equipment, intravenous equipment, ventilators, and monitoring) almost from scratch, and several notable pioneers have each contributed their own energies to this endeavour.

Very young children also have a unique range of surgical problems which are not encountered in adults. A small proportion of newborn babies have a congenital abnormality which requires surgery very early in life. For example, a baby with a severe cleft palate cannot suck effectively and therefore cannot feed. Even more grave are the infants born with congenital heart defects, whose circulation just barely works when oxygen is coming from the placenta, but struggles or fails when the oxygen comes from the lungs. A generation ago, the repair of congenital heart lesions became so successful that a cohort of such girls have survived into adulthood and are now embarking on pregnancies of their own, creating a unique challenge for obstetric anaesthetists: how to safely balance the

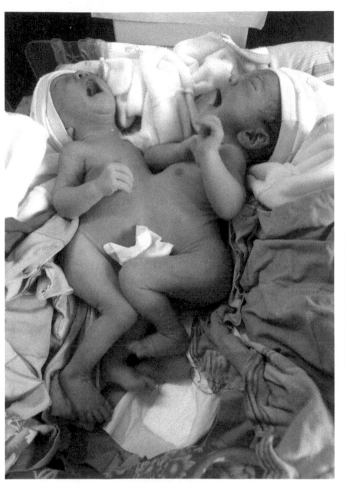

13. This pair of conjoined twin sisters was born in Hunan Province, China, sharing a liver and a single umbilical cord. They were surgically separated in April 2009 at two weeks of age and spent two further weeks in intensive care. Cases of this type pose considerable demands on surgical, anaesthetic, and intensive-care services

precarious requirements of the mother's heart against the demands of the baby during delivery.

Pain management in children has also lagged behind that of adults. For many years, it was believed that children felt pain differently to adults; in the case of newborn babies, it was considered that their demonstrably immature nervous systems rendered them physiologically unable to perceive pain. In those operations where anaesthesia was employed, postoperative analgesia was usually given sparingly amid concerns of overdosage. As late as 1993, a Canadian study showed that many doctors were performing penile circumcision with no anaesthesia whatever.

It is now established beyond doubt that babies, even very premature babies, feel pain, and there is some evidence that painful experiences in very early childhood can produce long-term detrimental consequences and enhanced pain perception. Techniques have now been developed to enable young children to communicate their experience of pain more effectively. There are now many effective analgesic techniques, including drugs and nerve blocks, to ensure children of all ages suffer as little pain as possible.

Specialized paediatric units and hospitals have elevated paediatric surgery, anaesthesia, and intensive care to a high level of sophistication and safety. Some paediatric anaesthetists practise exclusively in children, while others divide their practice between children and adults. It is recognized that, to maintain expertise, a regular commitment to paediatric anaesthesia is required.

Veterinary anaesthesia

Veterinary anaesthesia has matched its human counterpart step by step, with a rich and helpful cross-fertilization between the specialties. In many of the early experiments in anaesthesia, animals were used as the subjects, with the intention of human benefit. On the other hand, techniques and agents introduced for human practice have also proven to be beneficial for veterinary anaesthesia.

The *Lancet* of 1847 carried an account of the removal of the spleen from a Newfoundland dog under ether anaesthesia. A Mr Hooper of London devised an ether inhaler for horses, and published a picture of it in the *Pharmaceutical Journal* of 1847, together with some notes: 'In general the horse falls in about three or five minutes, when the head should be quickly secured.' One of the early difficulties noted in anaesthetizing horses in the standing position is the tendency for them to injure themselves when they fall unconscious.

A more testing case was reported in 1850, when a leopard in London Zoo sustained a compound fracture of the leg in an accident in its cage. Professor Simmonds of the Royal Veterinary College was consulted and decided that the leg should be amputated to save the animal's life. The animal was successfully anaesthetized with a chloroform sponge on the end of a long stick, and eventually made a good recovery. In 1855, an attempt was made to humanely destroy an elderly elephant with diseased feet using chloroform. The elephant was anaesthetized with chloroform but did not die until it was eventually shot, although it died without pain. In 1901, some 17 years after its introduction to Western medicine, cocaine was being used to improve the performance of racehorses.

While today the avoidance of stress or suffering in the animal is widely accepted as the reason for veterinary anaesthesia, and many countries have laws protecting animals from unnecessary distress, this was not always the case. Louis Merillat, a distinguished US veterinary surgeon, wrote in 1915:

> In veterinary surgery, anaesthesia has no history. It is used in a kind
> of desultory fashion that reflects no great credit on this generation of
> veterinarians...Many veterinarians of rather wide experience have

never in their whole lifetime administered a general anaesthetic in
performing their operations...Anaesthesia in veterinary surgery
today is a means of restraint and not an expedient to relieve pain. So
long as an operation can be performed by forcible restraint without
imminent danger to the technique, the operator or the animal, the
thought of anaesthesia does not enter into the proposition.

Sir Frederick Hobday wrote the first textbook on veterinary
anaesthesia in 1915. In 1919, the UK introduced the Animals
(Anaesthetics) Act, which made it illegal to perform surgery on
animals without general anaesthesia, and it was followed by
similar legislation in many developed countries. Debates still
continue about the amount of pain and suffering animals feel. An
injured dog behaves in such a way that it seems plain that it is
suffering, but the behaviour of an injured frog or fish or tarantula
is not so easy to interpret.

Today, veterinary medicine and anaesthesia are the equals of their
human counterparts. MRI scanning, renal dialysis, and
chemotherapy are among the options available to treat sick
animals. Veterinary anaesthetists have at their disposal the full
range of anaesthetic drugs and techniques, inhalational,
intravenous, and regional, which are available for humans, and a
few more besides. Some years ago, I was invited to spend a day
observing at a large veterinary hospital, and was impressed at the
range and quality of treatments available to animals. It seemed to
me that animals fall into three categories. First, there are farm
animals which are kept for milk, meat, or wool. Here, treatment of
the animal is pragmatic: if a sick animal cannot be quickly and
cheaply cured, it is usually destroyed. Second, there are animals
such as racehorses, which are valuable in a commercial sense.
Here, treatment of the animal is motivated by financial gain: even
if a racehorse cannot win another race, it may prove valuable in the
stud farm. Finally, there are treasured pets, when motivation to
treat the animal is love and companionship, and here the only
limits to what is available are imposed by the owner's ability to pay.

Chapter 8
Side effects, complications, and risks of anaesthesia

> Something that we were unable to detect was present. Something quite unknown to us that is capable of producing – let's call it artificial sleep. Now, that is a very remarkable phenomenon – quite inexplicable to us, and not a little alarming. Do you really think one is justified in airily assuming that such a peculiar incident can just happen and then cease to happen, and have no effect? It may be so, of course, it may have no more effect than an aspirin tablet; but surely one should keep an eye on things to see whether that is so or not?
>
> John Wyndham, *The Midwich Cuckoos* (1957)

The benefits of anaesthesia are so obvious and so overwhelming that at first it may seem unnecessary to consider its risks. However, no matter how benign, every activity carries some risk, and anaesthesia is no exception.

The impact of any risk can be considered to be a product of its likelihood (rare or common) multiplied by its outcome (devastating or trivial). It can be difficult for doctors and patients alike to judge risk accurately, when it is presented purely as a number. The patient might reasonably ask 'what does that number mean for me?' Published sources frequently show that people, including doctors, are generally very poor at judging risk and comparing the magnitude of different risks together, and often make emotional rather than purely statistical judgements of risk.

The most serious and feared risk is, of course, death of the patient.

Mortality risk

To be sure of the risk of death associated with anaesthesia, it would be necessary to take a large number of people, say, 1 million, anaesthetize them all for an indeterminate time, then allow them to wake up again without performing any sort of surgery in the meantime. A study of this kind has not been performed. However, one approximation to it is probably the study performed by anaesthetist John Lunn and colleagues in the UK in 1987 for the Confidential Enquiry into Perioperative Death (CEPOD). They retrospectively analysed almost half a million surgical operations during a one-year period in the UK National Health Service (NHS), looking for deaths within 30 days of surgery.

The NHS lends itself well to studies of this type. The UK is a developed country with a large population, about 60 million people, and about 2.3 million surgical procedures are performed each year. The NHS is responsible for the great majority of surgery in the UK, and NHS hospitals are reasonably comparable in their techniques and standards of care.

Among the half million operations, there were about 4,000 deaths, giving a crude mortality of 0.8%. Deaths for which anaesthesia was the sole cause were considered to be only 3, giving a rate of 1 death per 185,000 anaesthetics (which is a little over 0.5 deaths per 100,000 cases). A similar figure is quoted in patient information literature produced by the Royal College of Anaesthetists in the UK and the American Society of Anesthesiologists in the USA. More recent Australian data put the figure at 1:80,000, and Japanese figures are similar. Overall, a figure of about 1:100,000 would seem reasonable for the developed world.

However, this is not the full picture. According to the CEPOD figures, the crude mortality was 0.8% (830 deaths per 100,000 cases). Therefore, anaesthetic risk was a tiny fraction of overall risk of death as a result of surgery.

The CEPOD analysis suggested that anaesthesia contributed to death in a total of 410 cases, for a rate of 84 per 100,000 cases. However, although this figure is much higher, it is still dwarfed by the risks posed by progression of the present disease (which contributed to 67% of deaths), progression of another pre-existing disease (which contributed to 44% of deaths), and the surgery itself (30% of deaths).

A 2006 paper by Rupert Pearse and colleagues, based on retrospective analysis of 4.1 million surgical procedures carried out in the UK NHS, showed that the overall risk of death following surgery for all patients presenting for nearly all types of elective (planned) surgery is about 0.44%, or 1 in 227 (very high-risk surgery such as cardiac surgery was excluded from Pearse's analysis). For emergency surgery of any type, the risk rose to 5.4%, or 1 in 18. Further analysis identifies the risk factors of those patients who do succumb: advanced age, significant pre-existing health problems (called comorbidities), major surgery (such as major abdominal or chest surgery), and emergency surgery. Dying 'on the table' during surgery is very unusual. Patients who die following surgery usually do so during convalescence, their weakened state making them susceptible to complications such as wound breakdown, chest infections, deep venous thrombosis, and pressure sores.

This shows that, for a patient presenting for an operation, the state of health of the patient, and the nature of the surgery, are substantially more important in predicting risk of perioperative death than the anaesthetic.

The corollary of Pearse's figures is that, for a healthy patient having minor or moderate elective surgery, the risk of perioperative death (including both anaesthetic and surgical causes) is very low.

Awareness during surgery

Next to death, awareness during surgery is the most feared adverse outcome in anaesthesia. My patients ask about it frequently. Occasional reports of awareness are often widely publicized, and misleading statements about it are sometimes made, such as in the 2007 film *Awake*, which stated that awareness occurs once in every 700 anaesthetics.

Teasing out the exact risk of awareness is difficult. First, there is little agreement on exactly what constitutes awareness. For the patient, being fully alert during surgery and fully aware of the pain of the procedure is the most feared scenario. As well as the agonizing trauma of the event itself, it can result in powerful long-term psychological issues, including post-traumatic stress disorder. Most alarmingly of all, some patients in this circumstance may not be believed or understood when they try to describe their feelings.

However, it is accepted that this is not the only possible scenario. This is illustrated by a series of questions, known as the modified Brice questionnaire, first composed in 1970 to investigate situations of possible awareness:

1) What was the last thing you remembered happening before you went to sleep?
2) What is the first thing you remember happening on waking?
3) Do you remember anything between going to sleep and waking?
4) What was the worst thing about your operation?

Brice's questions invite the patient to remember going to sleep, and waking up, and then ask them to consider anything which they may recall happening between those events. The questions do not necessarily associate recollection with pain. The fourth question allows the patient to describe a recollection of pain but does not lead them towards doing so.

Brice's questionnaire still forms the basis of the study of awareness. It is recognized that the greatest likelihood of detecting an episode of awareness is to interview the patient on more than one occasion postoperatively, but the interviewer must be extremely careful not to lead the patient.

Studies of awareness have shown that a small number of patients may report a wide variety of recollections, such as snatches of conversation or music, sensations of pressure or pulling, vague impressions of people moving around them, or dreamlike experiences. Such experiences are not necessarily painful, nor even unpleasant, although the patient may be distressed by believing they were awake during the operation. Some of these experiences may have been formed during induction or recovery, rather than during the operation itself. A large recent study suggests that only one-third of patients who experience awareness recall any pain.

The medical literature contains several very large, recent studies of awareness. A 2007 study of over 87,000 patients conducted by Richard Pollard and colleagues in the US found that only 1 in 14,000 patients undergoing general anaesthesia experiences any form of awareness. Most of the cases of awareness were associated with major heart surgery. For patients undergoing other types of surgery, the risk of awareness was only 1 in 42,000 anaesthetics.

It is more difficult to estimate the incidence of awareness in children. On the one hand, their response to anaesthesia is different from adults. For example, children require higher levels of volatile agents to maintain anaesthesia than adults. This could make them more at risk of awareness. On the other hand, interviewing techniques in children need to be much more sophisticated, since children may find it harder to express their experiences, and are more susceptible to leading questioning. A large study from Australia carried out by Andrew Davidson and colleagues studied 864 children between 5 and 12 years of age after general anaesthesia. The children were interviewed on three occasions. Seven cases of awareness were discovered, none associated with any distress. This study and others imply that awareness in children is more common than in adults, but that children's response to awareness may be different from that in adults.

Causes of awareness can be divided into the following categories.

Equipment failure

Several categories of equipment failure have traditionally been associated with anaesthesia awareness. The first category is failure to deliver enough anaesthetic vapour, and includes the vaporizer running dry without being noticed, and inadvertent dilution of fresh gas with flush oxygen. Both of these are much less likely to occur now that volatile agent measurement is almost universal. The second category is failure to deliver enough propofol via a TIVA pump, of which the most insidious is an accidentally disconnected intravenous line. The pump appears to behave normally, but the propofol is slowly dripping onto the floor instead of entering the patient. A few of the early TIVA pumps had intrinsic mechanical errors which meant that they did not infuse propofol adequately, though these errors have now been corrected.

Human error

Error is part of all human activity. A typical anaesthetic requires the use of six to ten separate drugs, some of which need to be mixed or diluted prior to use, and most of which are indistinguishable colourless liquids. Due to distraction or haste, it is easy to draw up drugs incorrectly, or to administer a drug from the wrong syringe. Other contributions to human error include inexperience, urgency, fatigue, and stress.

Deliberately light anaesthesia

Three groups of patients have been traditionally considered to be at high risk of awareness: those undergoing general anaesthesia for Caesarean section, those undergoing open heart surgery, and those who are critically ill. In the first category, it was formerly believed that a deliberately light anaesthetic should be administered to the mother to lessen the risk of harm to the baby. This is no longer accepted practice. In the second category, it was difficult to administer a volatile anaesthetic agent via the cardiopulmonary bypass machine necessary to facilitate open heart surgery. More recently, TIVA techniques during bypass have become much more common.

In the third category, the anaesthetist may deliberately choose a light anaesthetic technique where it is believed that the patient's situation is too delicate to tolerate a standard technique. Such patients are usually at considerable risk of death, for example trauma victims with very low blood pressure. In a situation such as this, the anaesthetist is choosing the lesser of two evils: maximizing the chance of survival at the cost of increasing the risk of awareness.

Common side effects and complications

An effect can be considered 'very common' if it happens to more than 1 in 10 patients, and 'common' if it happens to more than 1 in 100 patients.

Common side effects and complications after anaesthesia include nausea and vomiting; sore throat; feeling cold and shivering; headache; chest infection; confusion; itching; sleep disturbance, and bodily aches, pains, and stiffness.

Postoperative nausea and vomiting (PONV) is a well-known side effect of anaesthesia and surgery. The main risk factors are known to be female sex, non-smoker (curiously, smoking is protective against PONV), a prior history of PONV or motion sickness, and intraoperative use of opioid drugs. Age of the patient, and the duration and nature of the surgery are all less important factors, although nitrous oxide and neostigmine have also been implicated in causing PONV. A person with all four risk factors has a risk of up to 80% of experiencing PONV; someone with none has a risk of only 10%.

PONV is usually treated with antiemetic drugs, of which the most effective are in four categories: cyclizine and other antihistamines, ondansetron and its relatives (which block a specific serotonin receptor), droperidol (which blocks a specific dopamine receptor), and the steroid dexamethasone (whose antiemetic action remains unclear). As with analgesia, the best effect is obtained by combining drugs from different categories. In addition, propofol TIVA is shown to have an antiemetic action. However, even with maximal therapy, PONV may still occur.

Sore throat is caused by irritation of the throat by airway devices and by cold, dry anaesthetic gases. It is more likely with an ET tube (40%) than with an LMA (20%), and least likely of all (3%) if only a face mask has been used to maintain the airway. Sore throat may be accompanied by hoarseness of the voice, and it is also common to experience soreness of the lips or tongue. Though unpleasant, these symptoms are almost always temporary.

A mild headache following any anaesthetic occurs in about 20% of patients. Potential causes include dehydration and caffeine withdrawal in regular coffee drinkers. The incidence of headache following spinal and epidural anaesthesia is 1 in 100 to 200 procedures.

Mild or moderate confusion following surgery is remarkably common. In the last few years, it has been the subject of considerable international study. The term 'postoperative cognitive dysfunction' (POCD) is used to refer to demonstrable reduction in cognitive performance (memory, attention, problem-solving) following surgery. Elderly patients who survive their surgery can sometimes end up 'not quite the same' afterwards, according to their families.

POCD is formally diagnosed by a series of psychometric tests administered by a psychologist. A 2008 study by Terri Monk and colleagues in the US found that POCD is demonstrable in surgical patients of all ages following major non-cardiac surgery. Monk studied patients who were young (18–39), middle-aged (40–59), and elderly (60 and over), and showed that 30–40% of all patients demonstrated evidence of POCD by the time of discharge from hospital. The groups were compared with a matched control group who did not undergo surgery. By three months, however, only the elderly group was statistically different from the control group, with about 13% of patients still affected. By about one year, the figure is believed to be about 1–2%.

POCD is not dementia. It is a measurable decline in brain functioning believed due to the effects of anaesthesia and surgery. So far, attempts to elucidate a single mechanism by which it occurs have been inconclusive, and it is likely that a variety of risk factors and intraoperative conditions intersect in an unpredictable way.

Uncommon side effects and complications

Uncommon events can be expected to happen in 1 in 1,000 anaesthetics, or fewer. These include postoperative breathing difficulties, exacerbation of an existing medical condition, and damage to the teeth.

Anaesthesia is designed to support normal physiological processes as much as possible, and therefore exacerbation of an existing medical condition (such as asthma, diabetes, and epilepsy) is uncommon. However, the stress response to surgery increases the propensity for heart attack and stroke in most patients, and patients with coronary artery disease or carotid artery disease are at increased risk of a postoperative heart attack or stroke in the weeks following an operation.

Some diseases run a prolonged course punctuated by occasional flare-ups. For an individual patient who suffers a flare-up a week after an operation, it is hard not to blame it on the operation. In the case of multiple sclerosis, for example, the evidence is that anaesthesia does not trigger flare-ups. The same is true for many other conditions, although some, such as acute intermittent porphyria and sickle cell disease, are known to be triggered by some anaesthetic techniques, and extra caution is required.

Dental damage requiring extraction or repair occurs in about 1 in 5,000 anaesthetics, though more minor injuries such as a small chip or crack in a tooth are more common. It usually occurs at intubation, although may occur when a patient bites down hard on an ET tube or LMA during recovery. The risk is increased when the teeth are in poor condition to begin with, or there are cosmetic repairs to the teeth: crowns, bridges, or veneers. The risk is also increased in patients with poor mouth opening or a stiff neck, both of which can make laryngoscopy more difficult.

Rare side effects and complications

Rare events can be expected to occur once in every 10,000 anaesthetics, or fewer. There is a wide range of rare events, and it is impossible to include them all. However, rare events would include damage to vision or hearing; life-threatening allergic reactions such as anaphylaxis; and permanent nerve damage.

About 60% of patients do not close their eyes under general anaesthesia. In addition, reflex closure of the eyelids, as well as tear formation, are abolished by general anaesthesia. For this reason, taping the eyes closed is universally practised; for longer operations, artificial lubricants may be deliberately placed into the eye first.

Harm to the eyes comes from two main sources; these can occur during any anaesthetic, and are distinct from any risks associated with surgery on the eye. First, abrasions to the cornea can sometimes occur, caused by accidental drying of the cornea, or trauma from drapes or other objects in contact with the eyes. Symptomatic corneal abrasions occur in about 1 in 2,000 anaesthetics. Although painful, they usually heal without lasting harm to vision. Second, an eye may be blinded by a process called ischaemic optic neuropathy, for which pressure on the eye, preventing adequate circulation to the retina, is the commonest cause. Permanent blindness is a very rare event following general anaesthesia: it has been reported to occur about once in 60,000 to 125,000 anaesthetics. Likewise, loss of hearing following general anaesthesia is a rare event; only 18 cases were present in the medical literature up to 2003.

Unpredictable life-threatening allergic reactions, called **anaphylaxis**, can occur under anaesthesia. A similar but less severe reaction, the anaphylactoid reaction, can also occur; in practice, they can be indistinguishable, and are treated in an identical fashion. Anaphylaxis to an anaesthetic agent happens once in every 10,000 to 20,000 anaesthetics, and is associated with a significant risk of death, up to 5%. The four main culprits are believed to be muscle relaxants, antibiotics, chlorhexidine (an antiseptic used in skin preparation), and natural rubber latex, although in principle it is possible for any foreign chemical to trigger a severe allergic reaction.

Nerve injury can occur as part of any anaesthetic. Under general anaesthesia, the injured nerve is typically a peripheral nerve, most commonly the ulnar nerve on the inside of the elbow. Injury is usually due to compression or stretching of the nerve itself, inadequate blood pressure during the anaesthetic, or both.

Significant nerve injury occurs in about 1 in 1,000 anaesthetics. Most cases recover fully, although in some cases this can take many months, and a small number of cases are permanent (fewer than 1 in 10,000 anaesthetics).

Nerve injury can occur as part of regional anaesthesia, where the intention is to block the nerve with local anaesthetic. This occurs in fewer than 3 per 100 nerve blocks, although the exact risk varies depending on the specific block employed. Almost all such injuries recover completely; the risk of permanent harm is between 1 in 5,000 and 1 in 30,000 nerve blocks.

The risk of permanent nerve damage associated with a spinal or epidural anaesthetic is extremely low. The risk of permanent nerve damage is between 1 in 23,500 and 1 in 50,500 procedures. The risk of paraplegia (permanent paralysis of the legs) or death is between 1 in 54,500 and 1 in 141,500. The risk of meningitis is about 1 in 200,000 procedures. These figures come from the largest ever study of severe adverse outcomes related to neuraxial anaesthesia, which was carried out in 2006 by the Royal College of Anaesthetists in the UK.

Risks specific to anaesthesia

There is a small number of conditions which are unique to anaesthesia, being triggered only by anaesthetic agents themselves.

Malignant hyperthermia (MH) is a rare disorder of muscle metabolism which is triggered only by anaesthetic agents. It was first described in Melbourne in 1960, by Dr James Villiers, who was asked to anaesthetize a nervous 21-year-old student with a badly broken leg. The young man told him that ten of his relatives had died under general anaesthesia. Villiers decided to proceed cautiously, but the young man became rapidly unwell with a high temperature under anaesthesia, which was abandoned. The patient survived.

In MH, muscle contraction is pathologically triggered, so that all the muscles become rigid, consuming large amounts of metabolic energy which is given off as heat. (A similar process would occur in a car engine when the accelerator is pressed to the floor but the gearbox is in neutral.) The heat produced by all the muscles of the body can be sufficient for the patient to eventually die of overheating. Injured muscle cells release toxic metabolites into the bloodstream. In addition, considerable demands are made on the respiratory and cardiovascular systems to provide enough oxygen for this hypermetabolic state.

MH is triggered only by volatile anaesthetic agents, and the muscle relaxant suxamethonium. In the absence of general anaesthesia, the patient is asymptomatic and typically has normal muscle function, although may be more susceptible to heat stroke. The underlying cause is usually a minor abnormality in a specific protein, the ryanodine receptor, within muscle cells. Several similar abnormalities have been identified, and the majority of these run in families. Most developed countries have an MH register of affected individuals, and close family members are offered testing. About 1 in 10,000 to 15,000 individuals is at risk of MH.

The mainstays of treatment consist of removing the trigger agent, actively cooling the patient (e.g. by packing crushed ice around the body), and slowing down muscle metabolism by use of the drug dantrolene. Unfortunately, when MH occurs, it still carries a 2–3% mortality.

People known to be at risk of MH can still undergo general anaesthesia safely, although propofol TIVA is the only reasonable technique. All local and regional anaesthetic techniques (for example, spinal anaesthesia) are safe.

The other specific anaesthetic risk pertains to the drug suxamethonium alone. Suxamethonium is a short-acting depolarizing muscle relaxant, lasting only 3–5 minutes. It relies for its short duration of action on being metabolized by an enzyme in the bloodstream (most drugs need to be transported to the liver to be metabolized). About 6% of patients have minor abnormalities in this enzyme, which means that suxamethonium will have a prolonged action. In a very small number of patients, 1 in 100,000, the enzyme is entirely absent, and suxamethonium will last for a very long time, e.g. 12–24 hours. Unlike the other muscle relaxants, suxamethonium cannot be reversed.

Routine monitoring with a nerve stimulator should make the anaesthetist aware that suxamethonium has had a prolonged action. In rare circumstances, it may be necessary to keep the patient anaesthetized and ventilated for several hours (e.g. in the intensive care unit) until the suxamethonium has worn off. Failure to recognize this condition (known as suxamethonium apnoea) could mean attempting to waken a patient after anaesthesia, who regains consciousness but remains paralysed. As with MH, a patient with suxamethonium apnoea is otherwise entirely asymptomatic, and may safely undergo general anaesthesia, provided suxamethonium is avoided. Patients with MH and suxamethonium apnoea are encouraged to wear a medical alert bracelet as a means of notifying hospital staff of their condition.

One final point is worth stressing. The risks of surgery in general and anaesthesia in particular have declined sharply over the last few decades. Surgery and anaesthesia are now safer than at any time in human history. Anaesthetists, supported by their professional bodies, have played a large part in shaping the safety of patients: recognizing sources of error, introducing new techniques and equipment, improving training, and designing better systems to reduce risks. In 2000, the Institute of Medicine in Washington, DC, reported anaesthesia to be the leading medical specialty in addressing issues of patient safety. Anaesthetists around the world are continuously working to make anaesthetic practice as safe as it can possibly be.

Risk	Verbal scale	Population	Example
1 in 10	Very common	Family	Postoperative nausea
1 in 100	Common	Street	Dural puncture headache
1 in 1000	Uncommon	Village	Corneal abrasion during GA
1 in 10,000	Rare	Small town	Anaphylaxis during anaesthesia
1 in 100,000	Very rare	Large town	Paraplegia following spinal

Very common	Common	Uncommon	Rare	Very rare
1 in 10	1 in 100	1 in 1000	1 in 10,000	1 in 100,000

14. **Magnitude of anaesthetic risk. In order to evaluate the risk of a particular event, it may be helpful to consider the number of people who must be exposed to general anaesthesia before one of them is statistically likely to experience the adverse event**

Hazards to the anaesthetist

When ether and cyclopropane were commonly used in anaesthesia, explosions and fires were a significant hazard in the operating room, and caused several fatalities. Since their abandonment, the anaesthetist no longer need fear being blown up at work. However, delivering anaesthesia is potentially harmful for the anaesthetist too. Studies in the 1970s and 1980s seemed to show that occupational exposure to trace amounts of anaesthetic gases was harmful, although these have since been discredited.

Anaesthetists work regularly with needles. There is therefore a significant risk of accidental needlestick injury with transmission of a blood-borne infection, such as HIV or hepatitis B or C, from the patient.

Some sources suggest that anaesthetists are more likely than other doctors to develop a substance misuse disorder. Compared to other doctors, anaesthetists have an increased mortality risk attributable to HIV infection, drug-related death, and suicide. Contributory factors include stress at work and ready access to drugs and equipment.

Chapter 9
Anaesthesia tomorrow

> The above examples illustrate the extreme uncertainty of any
> attempt to foretell the future. Potential prophets should always
> remember that a very numerous and prosperous tribe of
> bookmakers and turf accountants have for many years made their
> living out of this simple fact.
>
> W. Stanley Sykes, *Essays on the First Hundred*
> *Years of Anaesthesia*

With Sykes's warning in mind, I feel reluctant to make specific
predictions about the future. Anaesthesia is continually evolving,
and the next big thing turns into yesterday's news very quickly.

However, three particular trends seem highly likely to result in
changes in anaesthetic practice.

Understanding brain function

The human brain is the most complex organ in existence. It
contains one hundred billion neurons, interconnected by a
hundred trillion synapses. Faced with this complexity, it is likely
that our understanding of the brain will never be perfect.

However, imaging techniques such as functional magnetic
resonance imaging (fMRI) allow us to visualize activity in living

brains. fMRI measures tiny and rapid changes in regional blood flow within the brain in response to local activity of neurons, and does so painlessly and without any impact on consciousness. This allows us to determine which areas of the brain are involved in emotions, memory, arithmetic, and even complex cognitive functions such as the recognition of faces or telling lies. fMRI has been used to study mental illness such as schizophrenia, as well as pain states and the effects of analgesics.

Although it has limitations, and there is some legitimate debate over what it actually measures (blood flow around neurons, rather than the activity of neurons themselves), it is an enormous leap forward in neuroscience compared to older technology such as the EEG.

fMRI and similar technologies are very likely to improve our understanding of brain function, and this will enable us to better understand the nature of consciousness, memory, the state of general anaesthesia, and the effects of anaesthetic agents.

Working at the molecular level

Chemists and neuroscientists can now determine the specific, three-dimensional structure of complex molecules (such as the $GABA_A$ receptor) with considerable accuracy. By modelling the structure of a molecule on the computer, the interactions between it and other molecules can be simulated and predicted. In this way, for example, the way a drug binds to a receptor; or the precise way in which an ion channel opens and closes; or the configuration of an antibody as it binds to a virus, can be studied in detail.

The potential benefits of these techniques are considerable. In the future, it may be possible to design drugs that are tailor-made for a particular purpose, which may lead to new analgesics, new anaesthetics, new antibiotics, or new treatments for established, even hitherto untreatable, diseases. The only inherent limitation is the stunning variety and complexity of living cells, each of which contains many thousands of different types of proteins, lipids, and nucleic acids, all interacting in unpredictable ways.

Information technology

The widespread influence of information technology continues to influence anaesthetic practice. Like many doctors, my reading of medical journals is becoming less from paper journals and more from their electronic editions. My hospital provides me access to an electronic library where any copy of any one of many hundreds of medical journals worldwide can be displayed: this gives unprecedented access to the world medical literature.

My hospital has also stopped printing X-rays onto celluloid film. They are now captured digitally and displayed on monitors, which allows the viewer to manipulate the image digitally, to enhance certain features, or zoom in to areas of interest. The same image can be seen by any number of users, in the building or (theoretically) anywhere in the world. I can also attend virtual conferences, watching speakers from another city or another country transmitted over the internet. All this represents technology which is already commonplace.

I can see two main trends in information technology. First, miniaturization of components: my mobile phone can now store hundreds of hours of music and hundreds of digital pictures, as well as being able to connect to the internet, and in 2009, a mobile phone running chess software won a grandmaster-level chess tournament. An ultrasound scanner, formerly so large it needed a trolley of its own, can now fit into a unit the size of a laptop. Along with this trend comes the reduced cost that makes these devices accessible. Second, the increasing connectivity of computers and electronic devices: this enables the sharing of many kinds of information with almost anyone, anywhere. Issues of data security and confidentiality remain to be solved, but in the future, paper case notes, like celluloid X-rays, will be obsolete.

These trends promise exciting new technologies in anaesthesia, new imaging or monitoring modalities, and increased connectivity with mobile devices and wireless networks.

Anaesthesia tomorrow

Perhaps new vistas of understanding of brain function will unlock the mysteries of consciousness. Perhaps the perfect volatile agent or analgesic drug is just around the corner. Perhaps every anaesthetist will carry a mobile device with extraordinary connectivity and functionality.

The conceptual model of an anaesthetic 'autopilot' has existed for several years. If the output from a depth of anaesthesia monitor were fed into a computer controlling a TIVA pump, then in principle, the software could be programmed to adjust the TIVA pump to maintain the same depth of anaesthesia throughout. Such a 'closed-loop' system might eliminate the need for a human anaesthetist to be present to monitor the patient. The technological limitations of this concept might one day be overcome. Perhaps surgery will be conducted by remote-controlled robots, with the anaesthetic delivered by artificially intelligent software, and the patient will be the only human in the operating room.

But I doubt it. Anaesthetic care requires human contact: the reassuring and compassionate presence of someone whose sole purpose is to safeguard the patient's comfort and safety during the surgery. I believe that in the future, those ideals of anaesthetic care will prevail which were present from the beginning of the specialty: the desire to improve safety, to refine technique, to achieve and nurture expertise, and to alleviate human suffering in the most effective ways possible.

Glossary

action potential: the tiny electrical signal which travels down nerve and muscle fibres.

acute pain: the pain most of us are most familiar with; the pain of a scald or a sprained ankle. Most types of surgical pain are acute pain. 'Acute' refers to the time period of the pain (sudden and finite), not its intensity.

anaesthesia: from the Greek meaning 'without feeling'.

analgesia: absence of pain perception. Analgesia can be provided in a variety of ways and does not require anaesthesia.

chronic pain: refers to pain that persists longer than three months. 'Chronic' refers to the time period of the pain (long-lasting), not its intensity.

depth of anaesthesia: the concept that *general anaesthesia* is not a binary situation but part of a continuum from complete alertness to profound coma.

epidural: refers to the space outside the dura, the membrane that surrounds the spinal cord and brain. By common convention, it refers to the practice of inserting a catheter into this space to inject local anaesthetics as a means of producing *analgesia*. It is not the same as a spinal anaesthetic, although there are some features common to both.

ET tube: an endotracheal tube, one of the devices commonly used to maintain the airway under general anaesthesia. The ET tube is inserted through the vocal cords into the trachea, and a cuff round the tip is inflated, creating an airtight seal.

explicit memory: memory that can be deliberately recalled to consciousness, such as the tune of a familiar song.

extubation: the act of removing an *ET tube* from the airway.

general anaesthesia: a reversible, medically induced state of controlled unconsciousness intended to suppress awareness and recall of unpleasant stimuli such as pain and surgery.

implicit memory: memory that cannot be recalled to consciousness but which may nonetheless affect perception, judgment, and behaviour.

induction: the process of putting a patient under general anaesthesia.

intubation: the act of inserting an *ET tube* into the airway.

laryngoscope: a device for visualizing the *larynx* to permit *intubation*.

larynx: the cartilaginous funnel at the entrance to the trachea which houses the vocal cords.

LMA: the laryngeal mask airway, a versatile and useful device for maintaining the airway under general anaesthesia. The tip of the LMA sits over the *larynx* like a face mask sits over the mouth, hence its name.

local anaesthesia: the production of numbness in a specific part of the body usually created by injection of specific medication around nerves. Local anaesthesia leaves consciousness unaffected.

MAC: the minimum alveolar concentration of a *volatile agent* that will keep 50% of adults from moving in response to a standardized skin incision. At steady state, the concentration of volatile agent in the alveoli of the lungs approximates its concentration in the brain. Different agents have different potencies, so the MAC value is different for each agent.

maintenance: in an anaesthetic context, it refers to the technique of maintaining *general anaesthesia*.

modulation: the phenomenon that the intensity of pain perception may be modified by the state of arousal of the central nervous system. Situations of severe threat typically diminish pain perception, but there are circumstances when it may be enhanced.

multimodal analgesia: the practice of using a combination of different analgesic techniques in order to tackle pain most effectively, rather than relying on one or two techniques.

muscle relaxant: a drug that interrupts the transmission of signals from nerve to muscle, causing paralysis, which is desirable for some types of surgery. Muscle relaxants do not impair consciousness. (The synonymous term 'paralytic' may be found in the American literature.)

narcotic: in strict terms, a drug that induces narcosis, i.e. sleep. By convention, this refers predominantly to *opioids*. Colloquial usage implies a drug of abuse; I have avoided using this imprecise and unhelpful term in the text.

neuropathic pain: a subset of *chronic pain* caused by injury to a nerve or nerves. Neuropathic pain often has a strange burning or tingling character and is typically resistant to traditional *analgesics*.

nociceptor: a sensory nerve ending found in the skin and other organs whose purpose is to detect painful stimuli.

opiate/opioid: in strict terms, an opiate is a drug derived from opium, and an opioid is any substance that has similar actions without being derived from opium, or even having a chemical structure similar to opiates. In practice, there is considerable overlap in usage.

premed: a contraction of 'premedication', a drug given before *induction* to make the process easier for the anaesthetist or safer or more comfortable for the patient.

propofol: the most commonly used intravenous anaesthetic agent, suitable for both *induction* and *maintenance* of *general anaesthesia* (*TIVA*), as well as *sedation*.

recovery: in an anaesthetic context, it refers to the process of waking up after *general anaesthesia* is concluded.

sedation: a process related to anaesthesia in which consciousness (and often memory) are deliberately clouded during a procedure, but verbal contact is usually maintained with the patient.

soda lime: pellets composed predominantly of calcium hydroxide whose purpose is to absorb carbon dioxide from the patient's expired air to render it suitable to breathe again.

stress response: the whole body's hormonal response to injury and disease. Although its purpose is to promote healing and repair, some elements of the stress response are considered harmful.

synapse: the neurochemical junction between two nerve cells.

TIVA: total intravenous anaesthesia, the process of providing *general anaesthesia* using only intravenous anaesthetic agents.

vaporizer: a device which is part of the anaesthetic machine and delivers a specified concentration of anaesthetic vapour into the patient's inspired gas mixture.

ventilator: a device that provides artificial inflation of the patient's lungs. Ventilators may be used during *general anaesthesia* or intensive care.

volatile agent: a colourless liquid that readily evaporates into a vapour, the inhalation of which produces *general anaesthesia*. Examples include ether and isoflurane.

workup: the process of preparing a patient in such a way that they are in an optimal condition for anaesthesia and surgery.

Further reading

General comments

Specialists in anaesthesia can browse a very large field of literature devoted to anaesthesia, including half a dozen major journals, and many large textbooks which enjoy frequent new editions. Medical students can likewise select from a number of books aimed at them. For patients, or potential patients, there is also quite a lot of useful published information in leaflet form and online. However, scholarly books aimed at the interested non-specialist are few.

Chapter 1

The study by Ben Chortkoff and colleagues to investigate implicit memory is this one:

B. S. Chortkoff, C. T. Gonsowski, H. L. Bennett, et al., Subanesthetic concentrations of desflurane and propofol suppress recall of emotionally charged information, *Anesthesia & Analgesia*, Oct. 1995; 81(4): 728–36.

The same issue of the journal contains an editorial by Peter Sebel which gives useful background information about implicit memory formation under general anaesthesia:

P. Sebel, Memory during anesthesia: gone but not forgotten?, *Anesthesia & Analgesia*, Oct. 1995; 81(4): 668–70.

The reader will find a very thorough (though technical) description of depth of anaesthesia, implicit memory formation, response surfaces, and EEG monitoring in chapter 39, 'Monitoring the depth of anesthesia', in the 7th edition of *Miller's Anesthesia*, edited by Ronald Miller and colleagues (Churchill Livingstone Elsevier, 2010).

A scholarly discussion of the physiology of sleep and its relationship with anaesthesia can be found here:

M. Schupp and C. Hanning, Physiology of sleep, *BJA CEPD Reviews*, 2003; 3(3): 69–74.

A readable short biography of Arthur Guedel, together with many other individuals mentioned in this book, including Waters, Simpson, and Bonica, can be found in J. Roger Maltby's book *Notable Names in Anaesthesia* (Royal Society of Medicine Press, 2002).

Chapter 2

Anaesthetic history is well covered in a number of texts. Three recent, well-written books are *Chloroform: The Quest for Oblivion* by Linda Stratmann (Sutton Publishing, 2003); *Blessed Days of Anaesthesia* by Stephanie Snow (Oxford University Press, 2008), from which the Fanny Burney quotation is taken; and *Anaesthesia and the Practice of Medicine: Historical Perspectives* by Keith Sykes and John Bunker (Royal Society of Medicine Press, 2007).

The specialist may enjoy *Essays on the First Hundred Years of Anaesthesia*, by W. Stanley Sykes, 3 volumes (Churchill Livingston, 1982). Finally, the History of Anaesthesia Society publishes a journal of its Proceedings, all back copies of which are available freely on the society's website: http://www.histansoc.org.uk.

Chapter 3

More information about the role and scope of nurse anaesthetists can be found on the website of the International Federation of Nurse Anesthetists (IFNA): http://www.ifna-int.org.

A much fuller account of how patients of all kinds undergo anaesthesia is given in *All About Anaesthesia* by Jan Davies and Rod Westhorpe (Oxford University Press, 2000). The book is aimed at patients or prospective patients and their carers (including the parents of children) and is both detailed and non-technical. It answers many questions which my patients often ask me.

A considerable amount of patient-oriented information can be found on the websites of leading anaesthetic organizations. For example, the

Royal College of Anaesthetists (http://www.rcoa.ac.uk), the American Society of Anesthesiologists (http://www.asahq.org), the Australian Society of Anaesthetists (http://www.asa.org.au), and the New Zealand Society of Anaesthetists (http://www.anaesthesia.org.nz) have links from their homepages for patients and the public.

An excellent, short, readable introduction to TIVA is *An Overview of TCI and TIVA* by Anthony Absalom and Michael Struys (Academia Press, Gent, Belgium, 2005), but it is aimed at the specialist.

For medical students and newly qualified doctors interested in anaesthesia, there is much of interest in *How to Survive in Anaesthesia*, by Neville Robinson and George Hall, 3rd edn. (Wiley-Blackwell, 2006), which is succinct, amusing, and sensible.

Chapter 4

For a highly detailed and technical account of all types of anaesthetic equipment (laryngoscopes, tubes, monitors, ventilators, anaesthetic machines), I recommend *Ward's Anaesthetic Equipment* by Andrew Davey and Ali Diba, 5th edn. (Elsevier Saunders, 2005).

Chapter 5

There are several textbooks aimed at the specialist which describe anaesthetic drugs and fluids in considerable detail. Among these are *Principles and Practice of Pharmacology for Anaesthetists* by Norman Calvey and Norton Williams, 5th edn. (Blackwell, 2008). There are several weighty pharmacology texts aimed at medical students or doctors which cover many of the classes of drug used in anaesthesia: volatile agents, local anaesthetics, analgesics, antiemetics, and so on.

For a very accessible yet authoritative guide to pain and analgesics of all kinds, I recommend *Bandolier's Little Book of Pain*, edited by Andrew Moore and colleagues (Oxford University Press, 2006). Though aimed at doctors, the book is written in plain, no-nonsense English, and both students and patients will find it very readable.

The production and formulation of blood products may differ slightly from country to country. In the UK, the process of blood banking is carried out by the National Blood Service. It produces the

Handbook of Transfusion Medicine, which is available free online at
http://www.transfusionguidelines.org.uk.

Chapter 6

Once again, material here is aimed at the specialist. I recommend the
Textbook of Regional Anesthesia and Acute Pain Management, edited
by Admir Hadzic (McGraw-Hill, 2007). Hadzic works at the New York
School of Regional Anaesthesia (NYSORA), whose website (http://
www.nysora.com) gives detailed descriptions and images of a large
number of different regional and neuraxial nerve blocks. Equally
valuable is *Neural Blockade in Clinical Anesthesia and Pain Medicine*,
edited by Michael Cousins and colleagues, 4th edn. (Lippincott,
Williams and Wilkins, 2008).

Chapter 7

A well-written account of the history of intensive care can be found in
Anaesthesia and the Practice of Medicine: Historical Perspectives by
Keith Sykes and John Bunker, chapters 12 and 13. Another useful
article is 'The history of intensive care medicine' by Rajan Seth, which
is found in the *Proceedings of the History of Anaesthesia Society*, 36
(2006).

The website of the International Association for the Study of Pain is
http://www.iasp-pain.org. A lot of information is available there,
including a biography of John Bonica, though most of it is aimed at
the specialist. An excellent introduction to the biology of pain for the
non-specialist is *Painful Yarns* by Lorimer Mosely (Dancing Giraffe
Press, 2007), which uses amusing anecdotes to illustrate the
concepts.

The 1993 study showing that circumcision was being performed
without anaesthesia by some Canadian doctors is this one:

N. Wellington and M. J. Rieder, Attitudes and practices regarding
analgesia for newborn circumcision, *Pediatrics*, 1993; 92(4): 541–3.

A considerable amount of information for members of the public
about anaesthesia and analgesia during childbirth is available on the
website of the Obstetric Anaesthetists' Association (http://www.
oaa-anaes.ac.uk).

The study associating epidural anaesthesia with prolonged labour and instrumental delivery is this one:

M. Anim-Somuah, R. M. D. Smyth, and C. J. Howell, Epidural versus non-epidural or no analgesia in labour, *Cochrane Database of Systematic Reviews*, 2005, Issue 4, Art. No.: CD000331. DOI: 10.1002/14651858.CD000331.pub2.

Some veterinary history is mentioned in the history texts already mentioned. In addition, a review of veterinary anaesthetic history can be found here:

R. S. Jones, A history of veterinary anaesthesia, *Anales de Veterinaria (Murcia)*, 2002; 18: 7–15.

My own experience with veterinary anaesthesia can be found on p. 1262 of issue 25 of the *Bulletin of the Royal College of Anaesthetists* (2004), which is available on the college website: http://www.rcoa. ac.uk/document-store/bulletin-25-may-2004

Chapter 8

The annual CEPOD reports are all available to download free of charge from the website of what is now called the National Confidential Enquiry into Patient Outcome and Death: http://www. ncepod.org.uk.

I collected information about anaesthetic risk, including awareness, from many sources, including these:

K. Jenkins and A. B. Baker, Consent and anaesthetic risk, *Anaesthesia*, 2003; 58: 962–84.

S. Contractor and J. G. Hardman, Injury during anaesthesia, *Continuing Education in Anaesthesia, Critical Care and Pain*, 2006; 6; 2: 67.

I. Thomas and J. A. Carter, Occupational hazards of anaesthesia, *Continuing Education in Anaesthesia, Critical Care and Pain*, 2006; 6; 5: 182–7.

R. M. Pearse, D. A. Harrison, P. James, et al., Identification and characterisation of the high-risk surgical population in the United Kingdom, *Critical Care*, 2006; 10: R81. (doi:10.1186/cc4928).

R. J. Pollard, J. P. Coyle, R. L. Gilbert, et al., Intraoperative awareness in a regional medical system, *Anesthesiology*, 2007; 106: 269–74.

A. J. Davidson, G. H. Huang, C. Czarnecki, et al., Awareness during anesthesia in children: a prospective cohort study, *Anesthesia & Analgesia*, 2005; 100; 3: 653–61.

P. S. Sebel, T. A. Bowdle, M. M. Ghoneim, et al., The incidence of awareness during anesthesia: a multicenter United States study, *Anesthesia & Analgesia*, 2004; 99: 833–9.

M. S. Avidan, L. Zhang, B. A. Burnside, et al., Anesthesia awareness and the bispectral index, *New England Journal of Medicine*, 2008; 358: 1097–108. (Known as the 'B-Unaware Study'.)

C. C. Apfel, E. Laara, M. Koivuranta, et al., A simplified risk score for predicting postoperative nausea and vomiting: conclusions from cross-validations between two centers, *Anesthesiology*, 1999; 91: 693–700.

C. C. Apfel, K. Korttila, M. Abdalla, et al., A factorial trial of six interventions for the prevention of postoperative nausea and vomiting (IMPACT study), *New England Journal of Medicine*, 2004; 350: 2441–51.

T. G. Monk, B. C. Weldon, C. W. Garvan, et al., Predictors of cognitive dysfunction after major noncardiac surgery, *Anesthesiology*, 2008; 108: 18–30.

Major Complications of Central Neuraxial Block in the United Kingdom (Royal College of Anaesthetists, 2009). Available free at http://www.rcoa.ac.uk

There is an excellent series of patient leaflets explaining anaesthetic risk (including awareness and death) in detailed, non-technical language, available free from the website of the Royal College of Anaesthetists: http://www.rcoa.ac.uk/patients-and-relatives/risks

A thought-provoking editorial about anaesthetic awareness, 'I will be asleep, won't I, doctor?', can be found on p. 2120 of the *Bulletin of the Royal College of Anaesthetists*, no. 42, available from http://rcoa.ac.uk/document-store/bulletin-42-march-2007

A harrowing description of intraoperative awareness, written by a patient who is also a doctor, can be found here:

K. J. Rowan, A doctor's personal experience of awareness under TIVA, *Anaesthesia and Intensive Care*, 2002; 30: 4, 505–6.

Index

Index

Anaesthesia